One Small Step

One Small Step

The Definitive Account of a Run That Became a Global Movement

PAUL SINTON-HEWITT
WITH MATT WHYMAN

MACMILLAN

First published 2025 by Macmillan
an imprint of Pan Macmillan
The Smithson, 6 Briset Street, London EC1M 5NR
EU representative: Macmillan Publishers Ireland Ltd, 1st Floor,
The Liffey Trust Centre, 117–126 Sheriff Street Upper,
Dublin 1, D01 YC43
Associated companies throughout the world
www.panmacmillan.com

ISBN 978-1-0350-6504-2 HB
ISBN 978-1-0350-6506-6 TPB

1 3 5 7 9 8 6 4 2

A CIP catalogue record for this book is available from the British Library.

Typeset in Fairfield LT Std by Palimpsest Book Production Ltd, Falkirk, Stirlingshire
Printed and bound by CPI Group (UK) Ltd, Croydon, CR0 4YY

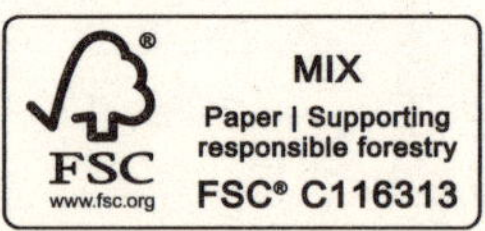

This book is dedicated to the thousands of selfless people who embraced the call to deliver social change to their communities, without which parkrun *may have never delivered to its true potential.*

Oh and of course, my incredible wife Joanne. None of this was possible without her backing, support and encouragement.

Contents

PART ONE

PART TWO

PART THREE

PART ONE

Bushy Park, Richmond, south-west London
Saturday, 4 October 2004
8.25 *a.m.*

When all is said and done, we just want to be happy and healthy. No matter what our circumstances, it all comes down to these two simple things. In some ways, they're closely intertwined. Our mental and physical wellness is the backbone of being human, after all. Sadly, either one can sometimes seem out of reach, as if they can only be found in some exclusive club.

Several times in my life, I have felt shut out in this way. Finding myself on the sidelines again, through nobody's fault but my own, I set out to get my own club up and running. This one would have no membership, I decided from the outset, and be open to everyone.

Standing beside the start line for my first event, which is really just the entrance to a small car park inside the grounds, I turn to take in my surroundings. An early morning mist hangs in veils across the park. We've had some rain recently, but this early in the autumn the ground is still firm. In the low sun under broken clouds, the oak and chestnut trees dotting the open landscape are cast in silhouette. So too are the deer herds grazing freely at this hour. But for the birdsong, the early risers walking their dogs and the distant sound of a siren that could be a world away, all is quiet and peaceful.

I check my watch. Even if nobody shows up for nine o'clock, it won't be the end of the road but the beginning. Should I find myself alone, that's fine. I'll be back next Saturday and every Saturday after that in the belief that word will spread. Whatever the weather, and through all four seasons, I intend to be here at this same time and place to host a free, weekly, timed 5K. It's not a race to find out who is fastest, I should say. Runners will have their own reasons for coming here, should any turn up at all. I just want to give everyone the chance to bring out the best in themselves, whatever that might mean to them. Above all, I would like this to be an opportunity for people to come together before the weekend gets underway and enjoy doing something they love. A run for one and all.

Just then, a squirrel draws my attention. It skitters across the wet grass, freezing briefly as if it's only just registered my presence.

'Good morning,' I say, hoping I sound relaxed and friendly. The squirrel observes me for a second before darting around a puddle and up the trunk of a nearby tree. When it pops out through the foliage on a branch, I can't help thinking

it's serving as a lookout for me. I turn to scan the pathways that converge on this spot. The mist is thinning, and though I see nobody making their way towards me yet I am so glad just to be here.

'Whatever happens next,' I say, turning to address my new friend, 'it's going to be a beautiful day.'

1

FIRST LIGHT

From an early age, growing up in South Africa, I learned that small acts could have big consequences. Take the fire I started as a little boy one dry, hot day in the early 1960s. Out of sheer curiosity, all I had done was drop a match into a jerry can that I'd found in our garden. Containing fuel for the lawn mower, and reeking of fumes, it was just there among the sugar cane that grew like a weed in one corner of the plot in front of our house. I jumped back in surprise as the liquid combusted. With a crack, the air seemed to split apart with flames that billowed upwards like some malevolent genie. Then, I had simply watched in awe as the blaze tagged the towering, late August crop.

I would have been no more than four years old. My brother, Timmy, was almost six. Unlike me, he knew how swiftly this could escalate. As the flames spread to the boundary fencing, it alerted the Freemantle family who lived next door and had been relaxing around their swimming pool. Even Mr and Mrs Cairns from the other house that bordered our place came rushing out. Within the space of a minute, I appeared to have sparked quite a drama.

'We need Dad,' said Timmy, retreating to the house as I stood there mesmerized by the vivid spectacle. A little later, even when the sound of the fire engine sirens closed in on our property, I remained entirely transfixed by the scene. My father had joined the neighbours in attempting to douse the fire with buckets of water, but I paid no attention to the adults and their panicked voices. It was the smoke plumes and the ribbons of flames with their ever-changing hues that commanded my attention. Even then, I had no sense that I had done anything wrong. I was just bewitched by how the simple act of striking a little match had ignited a transformation in the world around me.

Inevitably, once the fire was out and the fire crew had left, I came to my senses with a hiding from my father. It wasn't the first time and it wouldn't be the last. At that time, corporal punishment marked the tramlines of good behaviour at home and school. My family rented a house in Parktown North, a neat and tidy suburb of Johannesburg. We lived on a panhandle street from the main thoroughfare consisting of small, single-storey houses behind picket fencing. Our house was different. It occupied an enclave at the far end of the street, and was largely hidden from view by old oaks and jacaranda trees that bloomed with purple-blue flowers. A former farmhouse before the surrounding land had been sold off for residential purposes, it was an old ranch-style dwelling with tiled floors and a tin roof that amplified the rain.

I was the youngest of three siblings. Lindsay was three years older. She was quite the independent girl, and didn't share much in common with my brother in the middle and me. Mostly, this came down to us boys wanting to spend more time outside the house than in it. The plot wasn't huge, but with the house set back against the perimeter we made the most of the available space. With much practice, Timmy and I discovered that if we threw ourselves back and forth on our wooden rocking horse we could shuffle forwards. While it was always great fun to imagine we were cowboys roaming a wild expanse, I still have a little scar on my forehead from the time the front gate stopped me in my tracks.

It was a time of play, experience and discovery. As well as learning that matches were supposedly kept out of reach on the mantelpiece for good reason, I remember birthday parties and barbeques in the rondavel – a round hut with a conical thatched roof commonplace across the country – that faced our house, and the sweet innocence of childhood that once led Timmy and me to traipse to the local police station to report the theft of his bicycle. The officers had better things to do with their time, of course, but we believed in right and wrong, and so it felt like the proper thing to do.

For the most part, it seemed to be a happy upbringing. Only when I reflect on those formative years do I see the complete picture. In fact, the first time I sensed that family life was not quite as blissful as I believed occurred when my parents thought I'd gone missing.

My decision to vanish had sprung from a fear of being punished. My father could be calculating in how he disciplined us for any kind of transgression. Often, we'd be sent to our rooms before being summoned to his study for a hiding, and though it was administered with some force the wait was often worse. It all felt so unjust, and effectively just served to instil in me a sensitivity to fairness as much as fear. I grew to know when I had done something that would get me into trouble, but also when it felt undeserved. On this occasion, my father was out when I fell foul of some house rule, like forgetting to brush my teeth or make my bed. My mother warned me that she'd tell my father when he returned, which was why I chose to spirit myself away. I was very small as a boy, and had discovered that if I pressed myself into the corner behind the open kitchen door I could effectively disappear.

'He couldn't have gone far? Could he? When did you realize he was missing?'

It felt like I was there for hours. When my father came home, he found my mum, Timmy and Lindsay all looking for me. With my knees tucked up against my chest, and breathing quietly, I listened to the search grow increasingly frantic. Even the neighbours were alerted and joined in the hunt. At one point, my mother returned to the kitchen to telephone a friend. I could hear her moving around as she asked if they had seen me, and then start to quietly sob. This came as quite a shock. I had never seen my mother cry, in the same way that she didn't really laugh in my company either. Listening to her weep must've tugged at my conscience, because that was when I decided to make my presence known.

'If you promise not to give me a hiding,' I said in a whisper, 'I'll come out.'

The door swung away from me within a heartbeat. My mother scooped me into her arms and for a moment I sensed how it felt to be loved. She cried onto my shoulder before setting me down, as if reminding herself of some boundary between us, and then called off the search. I still got a hiding from my father, before being marched round to the neighbours and made to apologize for the trouble I'd caused. The punishment stung, but no more than usual and I soon put it behind me. But what I remembered most about the episode was the glimpse of my mother as I had never seen her before.

I was far too young to recognize that emotionally she kept us at arm's length. With no real understanding that she was more distant than most, it didn't seem all that odd to me when a work opportunity took her away for a year. She left without a fuss, and for some reason we children were deemed too young to understand. This would have been a momentous event for other households, where a parent engaged with her children, but for us it barely registered. As far back as I can remember, the family maid had raised us.

Constance lived in small living quarters attached to the house. A Black woman with a warm heart, through my eyes she lived up to her name. Constance provided everything from meals to kindness, and though my father treated her with respect it didn't occur to me or my siblings that her presence was a symbol of an unjust, segregated society. She had a family of her own, one she provided for but never talked about, and had travelled some 600 kilometres to work and live with our family. I hate to think about how she really felt about us. I have never been able to track her down to talk about those times and apologize for our role in keeping her from her family. All we knew was that Constance showed us warmth and care, and continued to do so when our mother returned twelve months later. Together with Timmy and Lindsay, we were thrilled to have her home. She didn't seem all that pleased to be back, however, and remained just as disengaged from her children as before. What's more, in the year she'd been away something had changed between my parents. They were tense and uncomfortable together. Their conversations would fall away whenever they realized they weren't alone. Sometimes when Timmy and I climbed trees or sat on walls we heard raised voices coming from inside the house.

By contrast, life next door seemed warmer. The Cairns had two boys of a similar age to Timmy and me. We often spent time together playing, mostly in their garden as they had the most fantastic treehouse. Constructed on broad limbs, with walls and a roof, this stronghold for the imagination was accessed through a trapdoor in the floor. Once inside, it felt like nobody could touch us. We had gathered there one day when somebody decided we should try smoking. We were all under five and drawn to the idea of playing at being grown-ups. So, having found some money in a study drawer, we took ourselves to a store on the main street. There, telling the storekeeper we had been sent on an errand, we bought ourselves a pack of cigarettes.

Back in the treehouse, in an atmosphere of excitement

and trepidation, we shared out our prize. The Cairns boys had a lighter, but just as we prepared to strike it up the sound of someone climbing the ladder from down below caused us all to freeze.

A moment later, Mrs Cairns's head appeared through the trapdoor. We were up to no good, and I knew it, and so I braced myself for the hiding of a lifetime. But instead, Mrs Cairns just looked around this gang of small children, cigarettes in hands or hanging from mouths, and nodded approvingly.

'I see you're going to have a smoke,' she said.

I felt my cheeks getting hot.

'Yes, Mrs Cairns,' I piped up, taking the cigarette from between my lips, confused by her reaction. 'Just one.'

Had I been facing my father in this moment, the rest of my day would have been spent anxiously awaiting a summons to his study. Instead, our next-door neighbour's mother considered me quite calmly.

'Well, that's great,' she said, before taking a step back down the ladder. 'You boys carry on.' She left just enough time for us to glance at each other uncomfortably, before stopping in her tracks as if she'd just remembered something. 'Just be careful,' she said, calling upon subtle but effective parenting skills. 'After what happened with the sugar cane, you wouldn't want to burn down the treehouse. Especially not while you're in it.'

Before Mrs Cairns placed a foot on the ground, no doubt smiling to herself, we had all returned our cigarettes to the carton.

* * *

When my mother left home for a second time, our father didn't even attempt to spin it as another work assignment. He offered no explanation whatsoever. Nor did he provide a return date. He just seemed derailed by her departure. In the weeks that followed, it felt as if he was there for us in body only – unwilling or unable to respond fully to the endless questions and chatter that children direct at a parent. In some ways, it felt like our mother wasn't the only one who had gone. As children, we just worked around it until one day our father asked us each to pack a suitcase. Constance helped, of course, but even she seemed strangely subdued. We had no idea where we were going, or for how long, but through our eyes it was without doubt going to be an adventure. We jumped in the car, sold on the mystery, and looked out of the window with excitement as our father drove us out of the neighbourhood. If we'd expected a long journey, we were surprised when, less than half an hour from the family home, he pulled up outside a big institutional building. Timmy, Lindsay and I looked at one another, none the wiser. Following instructions, we collected our suitcases from the back of the car and filed through the main entrance. Inside, a woman in a matronly uniform stood waiting for us.

Even before she greeted us, kindly but with a formal edge before running through the paperwork as our father committed us into care, I just knew we wouldn't be going back.

2

JAMES & MARY

My father was an outsider who worked hard to present himself as an establishment figure. James Sinton-Hewitt was born in Melbourne in 1929 to an Australian veteran of the First World War and a Scottish mother who had taken the unusual step of emigrating from a coal-mining village outside Edinburgh in search of a new life. When her husband died from injuries sustained during the war, she returned home with their son. As world events progressed towards another conflict, James grew up and developed an interest in photography. After taking an administrative job at a newspaper publisher, he was keen to learn more about an art that invited attention and respect, and so he persuaded the editor to lend him a box camera.

Shortly afterwards, on 30 October 1939, during a walk in the hills south of Edinburgh, James saw a plane tailspinning from the sky. Camera to hand, he captured a unique moment in history as the first German aircraft in the Second World War was shot down over Britain. He had rushed to the scene, not long after the surviving crew surrendered. The black and white photograph he took shows a crowd of locals gathered around the wreckage of the aircraft. It made the front page of several newspapers the next day, and would go on to be displayed in Edinburgh Castle as a document of the city's wartime history. It was also a calling card for the young man behind the lens.

After enrolling with the Royal Air Force, James served throughout the war as an aerial reconnaissance photographer. He was posted to South Africa, and when the conflict ended he stayed and pursued his passion for photography as a civvy profession. For an ambitious young man this was a country with boundless horizons. He established himself within an English-speaking community distinct from the descendants of Dutch, German and French settlers, a dominant presence known as the Afrikaners, though no less complicit in the apartheid regime that enforced strict racial segregation for Black South Africans. Within this bubble, James tried to build both a professional and a personal life.

It might be said that his haste to create a picture of success led to a first marriage that couldn't last. But whether too young, naive or hasty, James and the woman he married separated on good terms. Certainly his responsibilities towards a son from that relationship – my half-brother, Noel – added financial pressure as he worked to make his name as a photographer. Over time, his efforts paid off in terms of reputation if not income. With a string of commissions by the South African Tourist Board, he was attached to the 1947 royal tour of South Africa by King George VI. Such work came with social cachet and a source of pride, helping James to become a mainstay of the community that meant so much to him. He gave regular public speeches about his work and served as chairman of the local Rotary club.

It seemed he had made something of his new life. He drove a car that commanded attention: the oldest Rover in South Africa with 'suicide doors' hinged at the rear rather than the front that forced driver and passengers to take their lives into their own hands when climbing out at the side of busy roads. In keeping with his choice of car, James liked to dress smartly. He knew how to make an impression, which was either compensation or a cover for the fact his income fell well short of his aspirations. After the royal tour, commissions from the tourist board dried up. With no platform for his work, he was forced to move into contracted employment, which led to the occasional fashion commission.

Which is how James met a vibrant young runway model called Mary.

The photographs he took at that shoot show just how bewitched he was by her. With a biplane on a rural runway for a backdrop, the focus is entirely on Mary. Slim and toned, with long limbs and hair whipped up into a beehive, her natural, unforced elegance is strikingly captured by the man behind the lens. At the same time, he faced a strong young woman who had understood the measure of the opposite sex from an early age. On the face of it, my parents were made for each other.

Raised with two sisters in the Natal province to the south-east of South Africa, Mary summed up her upbringing as 'barefoot'. Born to Dutch parents, with little money to their name, she played football in the streets with local boys and was quick to get into fights with them whenever she or her sisters were slighted. In her youth, my mother had a commanding presence, and when that came to the attention of fashion scouts she soon found herself on the catwalk.

From what I've learned about my parents over the years, patched together from conversations with relatives and old photographs, Mary's career was rising high when she met James. She continued to model after they married and settled down, though motherhood would come to compromise the more glamorous side of her life. With two children in tow, living in a nice house in the suburbs that they could rent but not afford to buy, a sense of dissatisfaction crept into their relationship. As someone who pinned his sense of worth to material success, James could be unsettled when money was tight. It brought out his controlling side, further suffocating the marriage.

When she fell pregnant with me, at the tail end of the fifties, Mary made a decision that would have long-standing repercussions. One day, without warning, she took off from the family home, left the family behind and fled north-east to Southern Rhodesia.* Given the circumstances, it seems likely she ran away to terminate the pregnancy. Significant barriers to abortion existed in South Africa at the time,

* Southern Rhodesia would become the Independent Republic of Zimbabwe in 1980.

and though Southern Rhodesia shared the same attitude she may well have been able to make arrangements there. For reasons only she knew, however, Mary changed her mind. In any case, she chose to stay, which is how I came to be born far from the family home in August 1960.

Six months after the arrival of the son he might have never seen, James tracked down Mary. Somehow, he persuaded her to return and duly drove us back to Johannesburg. At border control, no customs officer asked to see any documentation for the infant in the car with them – which was a stroke of luck for James and Mary, as they hadn't considered that I was a Rhodesian national who required travel documentation – and waved them through.

My arrival marked a fresh start for my parents. With a daughter and two sons from this marriage already, it offered James the opportunity to at least keep up the appearance of a complete family. Mary may well have tried at first, but somehow it seemed she couldn't let go of the feeling she'd followed a fork in the path of life that seemed less fulfilling than the alternative. She was still involved in the modelling industry and was an ambassador for a fashion house in Johannesburg. Sometimes, she took me to work with her. As a small boy, I would watch the workforce treating her like a visiting princess; to me she looked like one too, as she tried out new collections for the designers. As a model she was captivating, in demand and under the spotlight. It was in stark contrast to her life back home as a mother, where she became increasingly disengaged.

Unable to let go of her career, and dissatisfied by the compromise she'd made, Mary entered a nationwide modelling competition. It was an ambitious move, involving a process of arduous rounds, but she could not ignore the prize: an opportunity to become a catwalk model in Paris for two years. As Mary went through to each successive round, the dream crept closer to reality. On winning the crown, which was quite an achievement, there was no question in her mind about her next steps. This was an opportunity she couldn't ignore. Perhaps James was reminded of the stories of her wildcat years in Natal, and resigned himself to the fact that she was beyond his control. It may even have become apparent to him that he had lost her as a wife. Regardless, he opted to maintain the impression that it was all quite normal, for the sake of their children as much as the world around him.

By rights, my sister, brother and I should have missed our mother madly. It's just she had grown so detached from us we barely registered the difference. She didn't write to us and if our father heard anything he chose not to relay it. Whatever strain he might have been under at the time, he had become a master of appearances.

So, when Mary returned from Paris a year early, James didn't celebrate her return or even seem remotely relieved to have her back. Our father just carried on as normal. Mary seemed flat, but he showed no outward concern that her experience might have fallen far short of her hopes and dreams. I would later learn that my mother in France reached the high life she had craved, and yet her work as a model almost certainly exposed her to the darker side of the industry, rife with drugs and coercive sex. Ultimately, we would never know the precise reason why she cut short her stay. While others in her shoes might have been reminded of the value of family, she came back to us as removed in spirit as when she'd left. As kids, we just didn't notice any difference.

By then, as James had possibly foreseen and even feared, the marriage was over. They kept up pretences for a year until Mary walked out. This time she left him with no story he could use to cover for her absence. For a man used to staging a performance, it must have felt as though the house lights had come on to reveal the set for what it was. My father's success story in South Africa was a fiction. He was broke, with a faltering career, two failed marriages under his belt and a total of four children who depended on him.

With nobody to turn to, and quite unable to talk about the immense pressure he was under, James Sinton-Hewitt made a decision that he must have believed was in the best interests of everyone involved. Experiencing what today we would call a 'breakdown', he applied to make the three children in his care 'wards of court', before then checking himself into a psychiatric hospital.

Like Lindsay and Timmy, I had no understanding of our parents' story at the time. As a five-year-old boy, I just experienced the consequences as we found ourselves uprooted from our lives and placed into a children's home.

3

SONS OF ENGLAND

The Sons of England Children's Home sheltered twenty-four boys and twenty-four girls. It was an institutional building tucked behind a suburban shopping mall, and worlds apart from each other. While one showed off alluring displays of the latest TVs and three-piece suites, the other was defined by two long and austere single-sex dormitories. The adults came in the form of matrons, cooks and caretakers, and all enforced strict rules to keep the place functioning. We could be kids, of course, but there were limits. Taking in children up to the age of twelve, I was the youngest at five. I was also small and slight. Faced with this strange, new environment, I felt vulnerable but also scared to show it.

Lindsay and Timmy must have been just as unsettled. From the moment we arrived, however, it felt like I had lost them, too. The girls were largely separated from the boys, and Timmy had just started attending a local primary school. Some of the children from the home were in his class, and so he quickly made friends with them. Before long, he was joining them in sneaking out to roam the shopping centre. It always seemed like a big adventure to me, but not one that I could share with him. Alone, I didn't know how to settle into this new life beyond just following the routine that structured each day. As a pre-schooler, that meant killing time playing on the trampoline with any other child who happened to be around, eating our meals at a set time in a big dining hall, and then learning to sleep in a collective space. It was by no means a generous, warm or loving environment. We were looked after by a matron and her supporting staff, but really they were just there to shepherd us through each day. Good behaviour was expected but not rewarded. Any transgression would be met with discipline, including corporal punishment, and so I quickly learned to do as I was told.

Being so young, I only saw the best in the other children. I just trusted them instinctively, and never thought that anyone would see me as an easy target. So the first betrayal hit me hard. It happened in the early weeks of our new lives. Lights out had plunged the boys' dormitory into darkness some hours earlier. With a matron at large, any early whispering had soon trailed away. Our beds were lined up in rows, with just enough space in between for each boy to have a locker to store his things. Having spent all day playing outside, I had fallen asleep straight away. Sometimes I would dream, which felt like a welcome escape. That night, there was nothing. At some point, I awoke with a start and immediately began to choke. In the gloom, I could make out a group of boys surrounding my bed. They were laughing. Some sounded gleeful. One was urinating into my mouth.

'Stop it! *Stop!*'

In shock and revulsion, I scrambled to sit up. The boys responded by laughing wildly. I began to scream, dragged from sleep into this nightmare, which was when I noticed that Timmy was among them.

'Boys! Cease this racket now!'

The dormitory lights came on to reveal Matron at the door. At once, Timmy and the other boys melted away to their beds. I was sobbing hysterically. My pyjamas and sheets were soaked. I was in shock, but not just from the humiliation. Above all, I realised that I could no longer rely on my own brother to protect me.

'Paul! Enough of this noise!'

Matron marched towards me in a way that stole the oxygen from the room. By now the other boys had squeezed their eyes shut, pretending to be asleep. I was beyond consoling. Matron approached my bed, her eyes narrowed, nostrils flared, clutching some kind of bat with a leather strap attached to it. Throughout my time in the home, the mere sight of that instrument struck me with fear. Somehow, she had decided I was solely responsible for the commotion, and by breaking the rules I was now in line to be punished. Bent over her knee a moment later, that strap stung my buttocks so hard it stunned me into silence. There would be no fresh sheets that night. Nor any sense that I was in a safe place.

Alone in the dark, lying in that soiled bed, I struggled

to make sense of what had just happened. Whenever my father had given me a hiding, he had first spent some time explaining why I deserved it. That had been normalized for me, but this felt completely undeserved. Traumatized, I tried hard not to cry in case it drew more attention. The whole episode felt so unjust, and it steered me towards a lasting belief in the importance of fairness in life.

I wanted to find Lindsay and tell her what had happened. It's just she was just that little bit too old and independent for me to feel like I could ask for her help. She had a close set of girlfriends, and might as well have been on a different planet. As for Timmy and me, we never talked about the incident. I was scared that if I mentioned it that might drive him further away from me. I never stopped loving him. I just wished I could have relied on him for a sense of protection. I was too young to understand at the time that my brother was also struggling. He was just another little boy in survival mode. While I watched him with envy, as he headed to off to primary school each morning, Timmy had his own challenges to face. Literacy was a struggle for my brother, despite his best efforts. It also singled him out for all the wrong reasons. Thrust into this new life, far from the safety of a family fold, he just wanted to be accepted. Unfortunately for me, the simplest way for him to do that was by joining the pack who picked on the easy target.

When I followed Timmy to primary school our relationship changed again. My brother had fared so badly in his first year that he was kept back and found himself in the same class as me. Even though my brother was dark-haired while I was blonde, other kids still thought we were twins and I loved that. Timmy, on the other hand, responded to finding himself boxed in with his little brother by firing up a competitive streak. If we played football or cricket at break time, he would insist on being on the opposing side to me. I was wary of him in the home when other boys were around, but in a team sport on the field we were equals. Even though he was frequently on the winning side, I just liked the fact that we were doing something together.

Despite the distance between us, we found an opportunity about a year after going into care to seek out something we all missed. Sunday school took place at the Methodist church beyond the shopping centre, and all the children from the home were compelled to attend.

The religious lessons sailed over my head, unlike the discovery that our mother had moved into a flat nearby.

* * *

Since leaving us at The Sons of England, our father had driven away from our lives completely. We had no idea he was in psychiatric care. For a long time, when Lindsay, Timmy and I talked about our parents we did so in the past tense. I don't know how Lindsay learned about our mother's whereabouts. Maybe as the eldest child, Mum had written to her. Having left the family home in Parktown North, she had resurfaced by moving into a small ground-floor apartment in the same Johannesburg district as the children's home. Her choice to locate there had nothing to do with the fact it was just a few blocks away from the church. It was just a coincidence we couldn't ignore.

On Sunday mornings, all the children from the home would be marched to the church as a formal group. After class, we were allowed to make our own way back. We knew we wouldn't be missed for a while, so we decided to make a short detour. As we slipped away from the group, my sister, brother and I were too young to feel anything but excitement. Our lives had become very complicated through no fault of our own. The last thing we wanted to do on seeing the woman who had walked out on us was make it harder for ourselves. Having learned that our mother had moved so close by, however, we just assumed she would want to be a part of our lives again.

Being the eldest, Lindsay was in charge. She led us to a communal building, and ran a finger down the nameplates beside each buzzer until she found the right one. When nobody responded, Timmy and I dutifully followed our sister to a side entrance and into a back yard.

'Well, hello!' Our mother was lying on a sunlounger. She was wearing nothing but the tan lines from a swimsuit and a pair of dark glasses, which she removed to greet us. 'You've grown!'

For someone responsible for starting a train of events that had led to us going into care, she seemed very casual about seeing us again. She was also completely relaxed about being naked. The yard was overlooked by several flats, but she didn't appear to care. None of us remarked on it, and I didn't think it was strange. As she was the only maternal figure we knew, I assumed it was all quite normal.

'I've just started school!' I said, eager to share my news. 'I'm in the same class as Timmy!'

My mother was smoking a cigarette, which she inhaled absently as if her thoughts lay elsewhere. Then, finishing a glass of red wine that sat on the table beside her, she rose to her feet and smiled.

'Who's hungry?' she asked, reaching for the gown draped over the back of her lounger. 'I'll make lunch.'

Had we returned as adults, the course of that visit would have gone very differently. As children, however, we were somewhat in thrall to this mysterious and somewhat magical figure. Mum fed us in her little kitchen as if it was something she did all the time, and then saw us out of her front door as if we were attending school for the day. She gave us each a hug and told us we could visit any Sunday if it didn't get us into trouble.

We deserved so much more from her as a mother. It's just our experience of life had left us none the wiser that her detachment from us bordered on cruelty. None of us picked over the visit on our way back to the home. We didn't comment on her lack of clothing or our wellbeing, nor the fact that she had refilled her wine glass several times during our visit. We didn't question anything, in fact. Slipping back into The Sons of England building we called home, before anyone noticed our absence, Lindsay, Timmy and I just fell into the routine expected of us. By then, we'd been wards of the state for well over a year. In that system, we couldn't make decisions for ourselves. Nor did we question anything. We accepted that most of our classmates were met in the playground after school by their parents, while we made the short walk back to the care home unaccompanied. We made friends at school, of course. It's just we could never be expected to be invited back for tea because we were different. All three of us lived regimented lives with no voice and especially no concept of what family could mean. There was little privacy, warmth or sense of belonging, but in those formative years we also didn't know what we were missing.

Without really realizing it, we had become completely institutionalized.

4

APPLES IN THE ORCHARD

Lindsay, Timmy and I remained in care for three years. As time ticked by, visits to see our mother became baked into our weekly routine. Over time, it went from a covert drop-in after Sunday school to a more formalized visit with consent from the home. Mostly we'd be there for an hour. Sometimes we would stay for the afternoon.

Mum continued to make us feel welcome. If she knew we were coming, we'd find her preparing lunch. Whatever had gone on during her year in Paris, the culture had influenced her cooking. A roast chicken was served as *poussin*, with new potatoes and salad, which became a firm favourite. I can still picture her at the worktop with a glass of wine and a cigarette on the go, which she always managed with some elegance. We became such frequent visitors to that flat every other weekend or so that Lindsay, Timmy and I even made friends with the kids in the same block. Some of the boys had gained access to a service room and refashioned it into a space for themselves. They were a lot older, but friendly and relaxed with us. One of them had wired up a record player and would play singles by The Beatles and The Rolling Stones.

It was my first introduction to music, and I loved it. Songs like 'Hey Jude' and 'Ruby Tuesday' transported me from my surroundings. That was invaluable to a boy like me. For the space of a song, I would close my eyes and feel completely free. Along with spending time with our mother, it was one more reason why that visit to her flat would be a high point in our strange, detached childhood. She never once talked about why she abandoned us, which is how we all came to see it later in life. When she mentioned our father, it confirmed he was alive and refusing to agree to a divorce, but nothing more. Despite what had happened to the family, somehow she presented herself as being the kind and loving one. Maybe it was sincere when we visited her, but ultimately when it was time to go back it marked the end of her responsibility as a parent. At Christmas time and other holidays each year, even if she was at home, we remained at The Sons of England.

While our mother's modelling career was on the wane, she never once lost her poise. That could make her hard to read. After so long in the care system, my siblings and I didn't question what lay beneath. We just took her at face value and behaved in a way that would please her. Conditioned not to challenge authority, we considered adults to be a law unto themselves. We didn't make decisions. They were made for us.

So, the day our father came to the care home to collect us, three years after dropping us off, he was met by children who must have seemed strangely subdued and compliant. In the time since we had watched him drive away, he had overcome the crisis that had hospitalized him. We didn't learn this from him until we were much older. Even without any explanation as to why he had abandoned us in the first place, we just packed our bags and climbed into his car without question.

Even though we were in the dark over the circumstances of his disappearance, our father had worked hard to restore some stability to his life for him to reach this point. Now he had returned to play a role in our upbringing. Dad had come to take us away from the care home, though the system decreed that we would remain wards of the state until adulthood.

Our father looked as well-presented as ever. In the three years since we'd last seen him, however, a great deal had changed. Perhaps recognizing that freelance photography could not provide him with a stable income, he had found work in the regional PR office with the agricultural machinery manufacturer, Massey Ferguson. His role involved editorial work for an internal magazine, which involved taking photographs to accompany the content, so he was happy. He had also ended the tenancy on the family house in Parktown North. In doing so, he had left the suburbs behind by moving twenty miles south of Johannesburg and into the countryside. It didn't take us long to travel there by car, but to kids with limited life experience it felt like we were entering a new world. As we left the city behind for what had once been a prosperous gold mining region, the transformation in our surroundings gripped our attention. The roads turned from tarmac to red dirt track, while the landscape opened up to reveal a scattering of farms.

Our father had reinvented himself to fit in by renting a smallholding. He came with no experience of looking after the land, and so it came as a surprise to find he'd taken on a place with a hundred fruit trees. They were laden with apples and peaches, all of which ripened beautifully but were never harvested. Throughout the time he lived there, he just enjoyed the sight of a bountiful crop and seemed content to just let them drop and return to the soil.

'What do you think of your new home?' he asked with great pride after we finished exploring. 'You're going to love living here during the school holidays.'

And that was the catch to what had seemed to be a day when everything would change. Our father had stepped up to reclaim responsibility for his children. He had addressed his personal issues and made a career change in order to provide for us. It was just that it had extended to securing places for Lindsay, Timmy and I to continue our education as boarders.

As my sister was at high-school age, our father had organized for her to start at a high school in a nearby town that housed and educated girls and boys separately. Timmy and I had been enrolled at the primary school just outside the grounds. Ostensibly a day school, here my father must have felt he'd secured an arrangement that would keep his three children together.

'You'll be boarding with the high-school boys,' he announced to Timmy and me.

As he painted a picture of this new chapter, no doubt with the best of intentions, the three of us absorbed the details in silence. We showed no reluctance or enthusiasm. Our lives were such that our feelings weren't a factor in the decisions made on our behalf.

I was eight years old when I moved to our new primary school, with my older brother in the same class. He was about to turn ten, but even that seemed like a generation apart compared to the high-school boys in the boarding house we joined. They weren't just much older. They were also more boisterous and extreme in how they expressed it. What was just banter to them seemed like a mean streak to a little boy, and it scared me. Even though I was used to communal living arrangements, this dormitory felt very different to the one at The Sons of England. Here, a long hall linked facing rows of bedrooms. Each room housed up to six beds, and seemed to go on for ever. From the moment I arrived, the layout meant it felt like I was being watched all the time. It also seemed very crowded, and I was constantly apologizing for walking into people. I'm sure it was designed to bring everyone together. I just found it hard to breathe. If there was little privacy in the children's home, there was none at all here. The girls occupied a similar set-up on the other side of the building. Apart from the dining area that linked the two, we rarely had contact with them. In fact, from the moment we moved in I barely saw my sister.

Timmy and I got along, but I knew that I couldn't rely

on him for any kind of help or support if I needed it. We were facing the same situation, and no doubt felt as vulnerable as each other. By rights, we simply shouldn't have been there. As the youngest in the boarding house by a long way, and still short and slight for my age, I stood out for all the wrong reasons. The older boys treated me with a mixture of curiosity and derision, all of which I just tried to take in my stride so I didn't make things worse for myself. But as time passed, the mean streak I had picked up on crept into their attitude towards me. Then it became cruel. The jokes turned into jabs and shoves, and the laughter at my expense grew louder. I tried hard to keep out of trouble. After school – where I had at least been among kids my own age – it was only a short walk across playing fields back to the boarding house. Even so, I would take my time. I felt safe out there, alone with my thoughts. Sometimes my attention would turn to the skies. There was an air force base nearby, and so I often saw parachutists tumbling out of planes from high above. Watching them drop was mesmerizing. They looked completely free from the kind of worries that went through my mind. And having found the courage to take the plunge, their canopies would always open to deliver them safely back to earth.

Compared to most of the boys in the boarding house, who had allowances to spend in town at the weekend, Timmy and I had no money to buy ourselves such moments of freedom. Our father couldn't afford to give us anything. We had each arrived for the first term with the clothes on our backs and a few spare pairs of socks and underwear. The house rules were very strict. There were places we could play and areas that were out of bounds, while everyone was expected to be well presented. As the rules were designed for older children, this extended to pupils taking responsibility for making sure their hair was neatly cut and tidy.

With no means to pay a barber, Timmy and I just let our hair grow. Other boys would often cut each other's to save money. We were too scared to ask, and even if we had it would have earned us ridicule or worse. In a way, being in cahoots with my brother who I so dearly wanted on my side, it all felt quite exciting.

For the first time in our lives, we were going against authority.

As the weeks ticked by during our first term, our unkempt mops became something the school could no longer ignore. We were told on several occasions to get it cut, and though we promised to do just that my hair at the neckline was beginning to brush the collar of my shirt. It was the headmaster at our primary school who finally intervened.

'Take this to the barber downtown,' he said, handing us an envelope after we had earlier admitted to having no money. 'And under no circumstances should you open it yourselves.'

Back in our room at the boarding house, emboldened that I was complicit in this with my older brother, I was the one to open the envelope. *Give these boys a short back and sides* read the note inside, which accompanied a crisp two-rand bank note. It was enough to cover the cost of two junior haircuts, but would also fund a decent haul of sweets. It was the first time in my life that I had decided to do something on my own terms, and it felt like an escape. That weekend, Timmy and I went into town with our hair blowing in the breeze and returned pumped up on sugar, additives and a sense we had bucked the system for the first time ever. We were united, even if only for a brief time. Of course, it earned us both a hiding. That came as no surprise. Every move I made throughout my upbringing came with consequences. But, just for once, that small act of rebellion made it all worthwhile.

* * *

Timmy and I spent two years as juniors in a high-school boarding environment. It forced us to be resourceful, if only to survive. My brother found it easier to steer a course simply because he was older. He learned to slip out with the older boys and then sneak into the cinema. On one occasion, breaking all manner of rules, Timmy secured himself a seat for a screening of *Dirty Harry* starring Clint Eastwood. To his horror, just moments before the house lights dimmed, he realized our father was sitting two rows back. Fortunately, the film was so engrossing that Dad didn't notice. When Timmy relived the story for me, gleefully spinning it as having got one over the old man, I felt like perhaps my place would always be on the sidelines.

Naturally, I wanted to feel like I belonged, but with all the banter and the bullying I didn't see how I would ever find my place in a group.

If it wasn't enough to be excluded from fun things because I was the youngest, I also found that it gave everyone licence to call me a weirdo. The easy target who could do nothing to fight back. It reached a point where some of the older boys would actively seek out a reason for picking on me, and also Timmy if we were together. This came to a head towards the end of the first term when they discovered that Timmy and I just couldn't cope with our laundry.

Is this yours? You revolting little kids!

According to boarding house rules, all pupils were expected to place their dirty clothes in a laundry bag. In order for it to be washed, dried and returned, every item had to have a name tag attached. This wasn't something our father had done for us. No doubt it was an oversight, but Timmy and I were too young to negotiate how to address it with the housemaster. Instead, finding a spare cupboard space in our bedroom, we took to stuffing it with our shirts and underwear, and even picking out items to wear again in the hope that it would see us through the term.

We shouldn't have to put up with this. Why are you even here?

Every single morning, the boarding house pupils would face an inspection. It was carried out by one of the older boys, who was appointed by the masters. Every boarder had a bedside cupboard in which to store our laundered clothing. We did our best to present our dirty stuff as clean, but inevitably we were rumbled. During one inspection, the boy assigned with checking our cupboards grew suspicious of the lack of clothes. On cracking open a spare cupboard door out of curiosity, only for our dirty stuff to drop out onto the floor, he transformed before my eyes into a raging monster.

Pick up your stuff right now!

Terrified by this sudden turn, which quickly drew more boys just looking for an excuse to torment us, Timmy and I were frogmarched to the bathroom with our clothes in our arms. I knew we were in big trouble as they swore at us and shoved us into the communal washing area. It housed a row of sinks, toilet cubicles, showers and a bath tub.

Drop your disgusting things in there, take off your clothes and get in, too!

By now, surrounded by a dozen-strong mob and with one at the door keeping lookout, I was sobbing with fear. These boys could have been ten feet tall. That's how small and powerless I felt as we were hoisted naked into the bath. By now, someone had started filling it with cold water. Another boy appeared with a whole box of laundry detergent. With great glee, he unloaded the entire contents into the tub.

Start marching on the spot! And don't stop until your filthy rags are clean!

With Timmy beside me, also weeping uncontrollably, I did as I was told. I could feel granules and clothing underfoot in the icy water as the boys ordered me to put some effort into it.

Whether it was a punishment, a humiliation, or both, it went on for ages. The boys took turns in standing over us, saying how disgusting we both were, and threatening us with a beating if we dared to stop.

We were powerless, and long after our tormentors became bored and drifted away we remained completely traumatized. We had nobody to turn to for comfort. My brother and I simply had to hold that horror inside ourselves and try to stay out of trouble until the term ended.

Then, for just a couple of weeks back in the care of our father, I experienced something I had long forgotten.

I felt safe.

5

ON TRUST

It was strange to see Lindsay during the holidays. Even though she was boarding in the same school house, it felt like she'd changed since the last time I'd seen her. My sister was no longer the quiet girl who put up with her little brothers. She had grown into a young woman with a voice and also a tendency to spark with my father. By all accounts she wasn't meeting the academic grades he expected from the school. Lindsay took issue, of course, and so when heat came into their conversations Timmy and I would use it as an excuse to find time to ourselves outdoors.

By now, our father had moved on from his smallholding. As if he'd woken up to the fact that the lifestyle brought little reward without the work, we found ourselves staying at a smaller, more practical apartment outside Vereeniging some thirty miles south of Johannesburg. While the city itself was a hub for industrial manufacturing, and the location for Dad's work, he had settled in a pleasant suburb on the shoulder of the mighty Vaal River.

There wasn't much to do in the apartment, but I would often find myself drawn to the riverbank. There, trees and bushes lined the water's edge. It offered a hiding place of sorts, and a chance to be myself. Sometimes I'd spend time there with my brother, but often I was quite happy to be alone. A broad waterway, the current was slow moving and serene. I liked the pace and the sense of peace. I lost count of the number of times I swam to the other side and back. At sixty metres across, it always felt like an adventure. I might not have been able to parachute out of a plane, but once I kicked off into the water, in my mind, there was no going back.

Swimming was one of many activities I enjoyed when I stayed with my dad. I also loved to ride my bike, and even became passing friends with some of the children in the neighbourhood. I had no heartfelt passion for fishing, but I frequently set off for a day on the riverbank with a rod and tackle. It felt like the kind of pastime a boy like me should have. A way to build structure and purpose into the days away from a school where I simply felt like I didn't fit in.

As each term passed, my defences weakened. I became resigned to the fact I would be picked on in the house as a junior-school kid in a high-school setting. Once, when walking along the hall to the recreation room, someone thought it would be funny to throw a dart at my back. It sank between my shoulder blades, and though I howled it wasn't something I dared to report. The boys knew it, and that only emboldened some to escalate their behaviour.

Had I found the courage to speak out, I might have put a stop to it. Instead, the targeting reached a point where nobody in a position of authority could ignore what was going on.

'Hey, Paul. Come in here for a minute, will you?'

I was just passing a bedroom when one of the high-school boys called me in. The door was open. He was lounging on his bed, while one of his roommates stood with his back to the window and looked on with a quiet smile. They were teenagers. Fourteen or fifteen at most. In the past, they had both been involved in mocking or humiliating me. It meant his relaxed, almost polite invitation jarred. Even so, as all the power and authority lay with them, it didn't stop me from doing as I was told.

'How are you?'

The boy on the bed sat up now.

'I'm fine, thank you,' I said, as he swung his feet to the floor and rose to his full height.

'So, we want you to do something for us.'

Placing one hand on my shoulder, the boy steered me around to face the way I had come in. At the same time, the other boy moved across to close the door. Each room along the hall featured a fan window above the door frame. It was hinged to open horizontally into the room via a looped cord on a pulley system.

The boy by the door began to feed the cord through his hands. Slowly, the window opened into the room. By the time he had finished, the looped cord was dangling away from the wall. I glanced back at the boy standing over me. He gestured at a chair in the corner of the room.

'Now move that under the window,' he said, calmly and quietly. 'And then stand on it.'

Something bad was about to happen. I also knew there was nothing I could do to stop it. Even so, at nine years old I was still young enough to feel that I could trust the people around me. So, after I had climbed up onto the chair, I didn't question what they had planned for me when the boy beside the door grasped the looped cord and placed it around my neck.

'There,' he said, standing back as if to admire his handiwork, upon which the other boy kicked the chair away from underneath me.

I can only think they expected the cord to snap. By the glee in their eyes, they were ready for me to crumple to the floor and weep at the fright they had staged. Instead, the noose pulled tight under my full weight. Hung from the neck, trying frantically to get my fingers under the cord, I flailed my legs while the boys froze in horror. It felt like my head and my eyeballs were about to explode. I couldn't breathe or scream, and simply twisted uselessly.

'Hold him up!' one of the boys cried, finally coming to his senses, and though I sensed some relief from the pressure as they lifted me by the waist I couldn't inhale until they'd finally slackened the cord to release me.

The incident lasted for ten seconds at most, but it was long enough to inflict physical injury. The cord had cut deeply into my neck from ear to ear. Lying me on the ground, the boys would not let me leave until they had staunched the flow of blood with paper towels and made me promise not to breathe a word. In that time, the self-assurance those boys showed on inviting me into the room had vanished. Instead, they were reduced to the same state of shock as me. As they begged me to keep quiet, it almost felt like I had the upper hand. I didn't want power, however. I just wished it had never happened.

South Africa is one of those countries in which every season can be hot. Even in winter, there's rarely the need for a scarf. Even so, the boys urged me to wear one around my neck until the wound healed, and that's exactly what I did every day throughout the weeks that followed. If I hoped it would help me to avoid drawing attention to my injuries, it eventually had the opposite effect.

'I can't keep asking you to take it off, Paul. Please hand me that scarf.'

It was my form teacher who left me no choice but to stop covering up. I'd been sitting at the back of her class every day, clearly uncomfortable in the heat but assuring her that I was happy to stay wrapped up. This time, perhaps assuming I was trying to disrupt the class by drawing attention to myself, she stood over me and demanded that I hand her the scarf. When I did so, revealing what I'd been hiding in a way that I hoped others couldn't see, she took one look at the necklace of bruises linked by a livid red line and the colour drained from her face.

In the corridor outside, feeling as if I had permission at last to cry, it didn't take long before my teacher had coaxed the truth from me. I had to repeat the account in front of the headmaster in his office, and when he responded by telephoning his counterpart at the high school I knew the matter was out of my hands. At first,

I was terrified that it would make life unbearable with the bigger boys. Instead, after measures were taken to discipline the culprits, I found some light came into my life in the boarding house. I never learned what punishment those boys received, but it sent out a clear message. From that moment on, rather than seeing me as an easy target, everyone just left me alone.

It took a long time for the lacerations to heal. Some teachers said how fortunate it was that the episode had exposed what had been happening to me, but I wasn't so sure I should feel grateful. It might have put an end to the relentless bullying, and yet the mental scars from that episode would remain with me for years. Above all, I found it hard to trust people. It went against my nature, and so from that moment on if anyone persevered with me they made a friend. Ironically, it was one of the older boys who made the effort. Clearly troubled by what had happened to me, Alan would join me at the dining table if I was alone. There, he'd just chat as if I were his equal and not some kid from the little school. Slowly, I began to respond until it actually felt like I could call him my friend. Rowing was a popular pursuit at the high school, being so close to the Vaal River, and it was something Alan excelled at. When he invited me to join him as part of a group, I jumped at the opportunity. I was too young to climb in the scull and pull the oars as part of the team, but I loved helping them to set up. Alan was one of those popular boys. It meant when others saw him treat me kindly they followed suit. I don't know if he was ever aware of the difference it made to my life at that time. I only knew him for a short period as he was in his final school year. Even so, I learned from him that compassion for others costs little but can be invaluable.

Whenever we stayed with my father, I chose not to tell him about what had happened. At the time, he was still sparking with Lindsay about the continued decline in her grades. That had led him to question whether Timmy and I could be doing better, and the last thing I wished to do was add to the drama. Dad wanted the best for us, but I suppose it was also important to him to be the father of three successful children. Even after his breakdown, and short-lived spell as a smallholder, Dad continued to invest a great deal of his time and energy in appearances. Having settled into his apartment outside Vereeniging, he became a regular at a nearby golf club. It was the clubhouse that attracted him more than the fairways and greens, and the *idea* of being a golfer. This time, however, his need to feel like an establishment figure opened up opportunities for him to build genuine friendships. He was a sociable man at heart, and this arrangement seemed to bring out the best in him. There were times when he also seemed happy away from the club environment. While he was no longer on cordial terms with our mother, Dad had always remained friends with his first wife. With a son between them, our half-brother, Noel, they made an effort to see one another frequently. Now that our father had a place of his own, he would often invite them out to the countryside. More often than not, and since his ex-wife was a wonderful cook, we would travel into the city for a meal at their house in Johannesburg.

Noel was ten years older than me, effectively a young man. The age gap meant we didn't have a great deal in common, but he made an effort to get along with Lindsay, Timmy and me, and I really admired him for it. Noel had just finished his studies and started work with the earliest generation of computers. When he talked about his job it sounded like he'd travelled to the future, and it left an impression on me. I certainly looked up to my half-brother, even if part of that was because his mother seemed so down to earth. She could chat and joke with Dad, and somehow they seemed like equals. I liked her a lot. She could be warm, funny and interested in us. There were even times around the table as we chatted, squabbled, debated and joked with one another, that I wished this had been my family all along.

6

THE LAST TO KNOW

In my final year at junior school, having put the bullying behind me, my confidence began to grow. I was still that small, quiet boy who could be wary around others at first, but steadily I found my feet.

I didn't shine in class as such, though I enjoyed maths and science. Just as I had a very clear sense of right and wrong, I liked the certainty that came with numbers and systems. Thanks to Alan and his efforts to involve me in rowing, I also found myself increasingly drawn to outdoor sports. I'd always enjoyed kicking a football around, but I never felt entirely comfortable playing in a team. Inevitably it came down to trust, which is perhaps why I decided that once I moved to the high school I could take up single scull rowing. I liked the idea of becoming dedicated to a pursuit, living the same lifestyle that Alan had shown me, and that gave me something to look forward to.

As juniors, rowing wasn't available to us. Instead, in my final year, I was introduced to an activity that would eventually form the focus for my sporting ambitions. Running wasn't considered a team activity at school, and yet come sports day we lined up as a group for a lap of the playing field. Standing among the school's rugby, cricket and football players, nobody seemed to be taking it very seriously.

On setting off, I hung back feeling content to just go with the flow. Then, to the sound of collective footfalls and heavy breathing, I began to find a rhythm. Within fifty metres, some had started walking. By contrast, I found myself picking off one runner after another. Steadily, more space opened up between the competitors ahead. I soon settled into a pace that felt comfortable, and just slotted into a position among the front runners. There was no real sense of competition, but in that short time around the field I experienced something that I had seen in the parachutists and imagined I might find on the water: a sense of peace and freedom. I didn't finish thinking I was particularly good at running. In fact, I was beginning to write off any possibility that I might excel at anything. Still, as I sought to catch my breath, a teacher made a point of congratulating me.

'Great effort, Paul. Really well done!'

I nodded appreciatively while feeling my face glow. Not only through the effort I'd put into the lap but also because it left me feeling good about myself.

In that final year of junior school, I had found some bearings at last. I was no longer just trying to survive from one moment to the next. I could see the path ahead.

I was also too young to realize that life is never that

straightforward. Having spent so many years inside a system, from the care home to the boarding house, I was used to having no say in my welfare or my future. It was the same for Lindsay and Timmy. Other people decided what was in our best interests, which meant we were always the last to know of any news from home that would have a major impact on us.

Dad had arranged to pick us up one Friday afternoon after school, so we could enjoy a rare weekend with him. My brother and I were excited. We hadn't spent enough time at the flat for it to feel like home, but we were looking forward to time out from school. With lessons over, we had packed our stuff and were ready to go. Other boarders often went home at the end of each week, so it felt like a transition was underway.

One hour after the last boy had left, telling us he'd see us on Sunday, it became clear that our father wasn't coming for us.

Naturally, Timmy and I were disappointed. Even so, we didn't ask why he hadn't shown up. Nor did we try to track down Lindsay, who we saw so rarely anyway. We just went back to our rooms, unpacked our bags and got on with our weekend.

The following Friday, as a few boys prepared to head home once again, a familiar figure came to collect us. It wasn't our father, but a colleague of his from work. The pair were friends, and we had met him once when he visited the country club.

'My wife and I thought you'd like a break,' he said, having come to collect their two sons who also attended the school.

We were all of a similar age, and got along fine, and so

it seemed like quite a treat. Timmy and I set out to make the most of being part of a family for the weekend, and read nothing into the lingering looks that the other boys' parents levelled at us. It was odd, but we were just happy to be away from school.

A week later, much to our surprise, our stepbrother arrived to bring us home.

It was always good to see Noel, though he seemed subdued as we expressed surprise and excitement at his appearance at the school.

'Your mum is waiting in the car for us,' he said, which silenced us both.

We hadn't seen or heard from our mother since leaving the children's home. Not only that but we thought of our stepbrother as belonging to another side of our fractured family. To learn that the pair had travelled here together was both surprising and a little alarming. Sensing that all was not well, we followed Noel into the school car park.

Our mother was standing with her back to the passenger door, smoking the last of a cigarette. Lindsay was already in the back seat. She was drying her eyes, I realized.

'Boys,' said Mum, stamping out the stub with the heel of her shoe. 'I have some news . . .'

My father rarely attended the golf club to play a round. Mostly, he spent time there to socialize at the bar. He enjoyed the company of the players, and the sense of camaraderie they brought back from the fairways. The night before he had been due to collect us from school for the weekend, he made too much of that spirit and set off for home in his car some way over the drink-driving limit. Shortly after leaving the club, he'd been lucky to escape with his life on speeding into a crash of his own making.

The accident involved no other road users, but left our father with serious head injuries. He had been in a coma at the hospital, we learned as our mother explained the situation and Noel drove us there. While he had now stabilized, she told us, for some time there had been a chance he wouldn't pull through.

'Why didn't anyone tell us?' asked Timmy at one point.

From the passenger seat, our mother had been turning to address us as she shared the news. This time, she just didn't seem to register the question.

'Noel has been amazing,' she said. 'He's made arrangements to look after your dad when he comes home.'

'It'll be some time yet,' my stepbrother added. 'But we're hopeful.'

On waiting to see Dad, our sense of shock seemed misplaced. The accident had happened weeks ago, and though he'd been left with serious injuries his life was no longer in danger. We waited in the corridor with Noel as our mother went in first. I noticed she had a manilla envelope with her which contained some documents.

'What's that for?' I asked our stepbrother.

'Some admin,' he offered without looking at me, and then appeared to reconsider his answer. My brother and I were sitting on plastic chairs under the window. Lindsay was pacing the floor, but soon gravitated closer when Noel crouched before us.

'We all know your mother has been asking for a divorce for some time,' he said, and we nodded because in her flat she had often complained that our father refused. 'Well, she's here so he can sign the papers.'

The three of us absorbed the news in silence. It seemed far less important than the fact that we'd nearly lost him altogether.

A few minutes later, when our mother emerged from his room, she seemed happier to see us than she had when we came out of school.

'It's so good to see you again,' she cooed, hugging us in turn before tucking the envelope into her handbag. 'I'm sure your dad will be just as pleased.'

When our time came, Noel led us to his bedside. We filed in without word, and just took a moment to absorb the stillness in the room. Our father's eyes were closed, but I had to register his chest rise and fall to be sure he was even alive. His throat was heavily bandaged, and we learned that until recently he had been breathing through tracheotomy tubes. He was in a terrible state, and it seemed far worse than anyone had described so far.

'Dad . . .'

Lindsay took the seat that our mother must have drawn up beside his bed. She clasped his hand and held it in hers. In response, our father opened his eyes. He smiled weakly before his lids closed once again. I glanced at Timmy. Like me, as our sister wept, my brother seemed to be fully focused on holding his composure. I just didn't know how to process what had happened. Nobody was on hand to reassure me that my response, whatever that might be, was fine. Thinking I shouldn't add to the tears, I stared at the fold in the bedsheet across his chest in a bid to hold on. I noticed a pen in the spot where his hand had been resting, which Noel quietly removed as if perhaps we might dwell on how a man in his condition was capable of writing his signature without assistance.

In the weeks and months that followed, it was Noel who held the family together. Lindsay, Timmy and I returned to school, but now our stepbrother appeared to have the authority to keep us in the picture. He worked really hard to spin all the plates, holding down his job as a computer programmer while stepping into the role of carer when our father was finally discharged from hospital. Our mother hung around for a while. She made a great deal of noise about helping out, but it was all words and little action. She had started seeing a new man, as she told us with great enthusiasm; an estate agent from Johannesburg called Roger who drove an Audi Quatro. When she introduced us to him, he struck me as someone who had fallen for our mother's beauty and accepted it was only skin deep. He seemed to turn a blind eye to her track record as a mother, and knew how to impress her with his flash car and a nice house that she would share with him until they split several years later. While we were pleased to see her looking happy, it was also enough for us to think she was set to vanish from our lives once again.

As we finished our final term at school, Noel took out a mortgage on a small place in Johannesburg that would allow our father to move in with him. The flat outside Vereeniging was no longer practical. It was just too far away for my stepbrother who had to juggle work with his new responsibility as a carer. The injury to Dad's brain had resulted in a loss of feeling down much of the left-hand side of his body. He couldn't walk without assistance and only had the use of one arm. The doctors stressed that he faced a long road to recovery, cautioning that he would be reliant on others for a long time to come. Having moved Dad into the new place, Noel would make every effort to bring us back from school to visit him at weekends.

'He might not be able to show it,' he told us, 'but it means a lot to him to see you all.'

I had just turned twelve. I was finally growing, and yet it still felt like the rest of my class had left me behind. On spending time with our father, however, I began to feel like I was the adult. The brain injury seemed to slow his thoughts and actions. Spending most of his days in an armchair, our father was entirely dependent on Noel to go to the bathroom or feed himself. When I talked to him, which our stepbrother encouraged us to do, I was often met by a glassy stare that made me wonder if he was registering anything that I said. He still looked like my dad, even if he'd lost a lot of weight, but now there was an air of vulnerability about him. For a man who used to instil discipline in his children with a careful, considered use of the belt, it was as though he had lost all authority.

At least, it seemed that way until we learned that before his accident our father had made another big decision about our future.

It was Lindsay's poor academic performance that had persuaded him to move us all to another school. According to Noel, Dad had convinced himself that Timmy and I would let ourselves down if we stayed. As a result, based on recommendation from friends who had made a success of their lives, he secured places for my sister, my brother and me at another boarding school in the university town of Potchefstroom. It was over a hundred kilometres away to the south-east, and none of us knew anybody there. Even if our father had been well, I doubt that Timmy or I would have put up any resistance. I didn't want to leave. It had taken me years to finally feel settled, and this move would scupper my dreams of becoming a rower. I also knew that I had no say in the matter. Given his frail condition, even Lindsay seemed to accept that there would be no conversation or negotiation to be had about the situation. Come the new term we would just move on to another phase in the system that had overseen our lives so far.

7

THE BALANCE OF POWER

Potchefstroom High School, known as Potch by everyone from the headmaster down, was quite literally in a class of its own. One of the oldest schools in South Africa, established in 1905, much of its character was modelled on classic English educational establishments. Before the new term started, Noel took us shopping for uniforms and the various compulsory items we had to bring as pupils.

'What do you think?' I asked Timmy at the store, as I tried on the blazer, tie and boater we were expected to wear.

'Posh!' he said. 'A posh clown.'

Normally, our father wouldn't tolerate this kind of exchange. Noel had brought him with us in a wheelchair, which at least prevented him from being completely house-bound. But instead of reprimanding Timmy he just watched impassively as we larked around. Even Lindsay found it hard to take the dress code seriously, though when Noel became tired of the joking around we focused on the task at hand. None of us had asked to be in this situation, but we respected the fact that our stepbrother was sacrificing a great deal to keep our family functioning.

When the new term started, reality set in hard. What had felt like fancy dress became the clothes we were expected to wear every day. It wasn't an expensive fee-paying school populated by the children of the rich and elite. Potch just maintained standards in everything from dress code to the quality of teaching and pupil behaviour. Set in the heart of huge grounds, the school comprised of a series of white single-storey buildings with red rooftops bordering courtyards that could have been copied and pasted from Oxford or Cambridge. Founded more than one hundred years earlier, Potch was certainly rich in tradition. It's just through my eyes some of the old ways didn't seem to be in the best interests of the pupils.

Having spent several years in a boarders' house, Timmy and I did at least find some elements of our transition to high school to be relatively straightforward. We'd lived away from home for much of our lives, and almost always as the youngest in a group. Once again, boys and girls were housed and educated separately, which meant Lindsay effectively vanished. While other boys in their first year seemed quite fragile to begin with, missing their parents or the comforts of home, we knew that submitting to the new rules and regulations was the easiest way to function. As well-oiled cogs in a big machine, we knew that if we showed any kind of resistance it would only break us.

What came as a surprise to Timmy and me in this system was that the youngest pupils were expected to run errands and domestic duties for the seniors. It was supposed to be restricted to tidying rooms, shining shoes and making cups of tea. Even as an age-old custom, it didn't take long for me to realize it could be grossly unfair and open to abuse. First-year pupils like me could find ourselves ordered about at a moment's notice, and treated with a mixture of contempt, mockery and aggression based solely on the fact that those in power were older and physically bigger than us.

'Pack my school bag every day,' said the sixth-former I had been allocated to serve. He had only just started to run through the list of tasks I was expected to carry out for him. Already this seemed quite enough. 'That means going through my timetable and making sure I have all the right textbooks.'

He didn't need to spell out the consequences if I made a mistake. I was used to reading veiled threats from tone and body language alone. It meant every morning I had to get up early to tidy his room while he showered, make his bed and lay out his uniform for the day. On my first attempt, quite possibly so he could impress his roommates, he determined that the crease in the bed sheets wasn't sharp enough. Finishing his inspection, in front of several other sixth-formers, he turned and struck the side of my head with one hand. From that moment on, in a role that would last an entire academic year, I set out to give him no further reason to hurt me. I found that as long as I did everything right, he treated me fairly.

Other boys weren't so fortunate. Even if they made no

mistakes in their duties, they were regularly punished for their efforts. Distressingly, it was Timmy who suffered more than anyone else. He'd been allocated to a sixth-former with a sadistic streak. It didn't help that the boy's roommates encouraged him in the beatings that my brother suffered throughout that year, and sometimes even joined in. Even though my brother had taken sides against me in the past, I hated to see him go through a similar experience. Like him, I'd just learned to soak up the violence and humiliation. We'd grown up without a parent or adult who could step in on our behalf. As much as I wanted to stand up for Timmy, I was still just a little kid to the older boys. I didn't want to abandon my brother because I knew how that felt. All I could do was ask him if he needed anything whenever I found him weeping or alone. He'd often send me packing, but it felt like the right thing to do.

Like all first-year pupils, I found it hard to escape from the constant threat that something bad would happen. We were on call to sixth-formers and prefects, many of whom used intimidation and violence without warning. At any time, I could be called out to make a cup of tea or fold away clothes, which just left me feeling anxious and on edge. With no permission to leave school grounds, we had nowhere to hide. Even so, I still discovered a form of escape that I would turn to throughout my education. Radio became a friend to me that I could trust. I had a little portable device that Noel's mother had given me on a visit to her house one holiday. Every evening, I would lie on my bed with it resting on my pillow and explore the airwaves. Music fascinated me, especially if I could close my eyes and let it transport me in my imagination. I still loved The Beatles and The Rolling Stones, but also found myself drawn to a lot of rock music that the other boys liked such as Black Sabbath and Pink Floyd.

On Friday evenings, turning through the dial, I found a police drama series. It would bring me back at the same time every week for the next instalment. With each episode that aired, I found my roommates drawing close so they could listen in too. It became a shared experience, and when the batteries ran out I was undeterred. With no money to replace them, or much care about my safety, I decided to copy a trick I'd seen one of the sixth-formers perform with the light socket in his room. I removed the bulb and smashed the glass to reveal the electrodes. Then, using an electrical cord, a strip of tape and some intervention from a roommate who claimed I would otherwise electrocute myself, we managed to hook up the radio to the mains without frying ourselves. It was stupidly dangerous, but also thrilling, and made our cop show sessions all the more rewarding. For half an hour every week, we were no longer meek first years seeking a moment away from our tormentors, but crime fighters on the mean and dirty streets.

At the end of that first year, on being released from what was effectively a campaign of licensed bullying, life at Potch improved a little. The radio sessions had helped me to make a few friends in my year. Like me, they were quiet and preferred to be on the edge of things. We certainly weren't considered to be among the popular boys. It meant the threat of a beating never completely went away. It was as if the sixth-formers had become drunk on their own power, and set out to dominate every year below them. Over time, it left me with nothing but disdain for those jocks who sought to make themselves feel big by picking on those who were smaller, weaker or defenceless. On the playing fields one day, during a game of cricket, I congratulated a friend who had hit a winning six by rushing across to hug him. In the excitement of the moment, it seemed like a perfectly normal thing to do on the field. For a group of older boys who were watching from the dorm window, however, it was an offence that merited a summons. In their room later that day, having been mocked for behaving 'like a pansy', I was ordered to submit to a savage battering with a hockey stick that left me bruised and shaken. I grew to loathe that kind of behaviour. In a system that encouraged abuse, I had no desire to follow in their footsteps as I moved up through the school.

Emotionally, it felt like I was growing up faster than those who delighted on picking on others. Boys several years above would act in ways that made me think of them as immature kids. As I continued to develop physically their attitude towards me changed. On turning fourteen, I experienced another growth spurt that saw me go from being one of the smallest in my class to the tallest. Older boys who had previously picked on me began to leave me alone. I was by no means immune from being threatened with a kicking for some perceived slight, but from that moment on my life at school became a little more bearable.

It took a while for me to feel comfortable with adolescence. I was used to being the small, weedy kid, and now I towered above so many of my friends. I was still slim-built, but somehow found it harder to keep my head down.

It didn't bring me much confidence at school. On visiting my father, however, the physical contrast between us emboldened me. As a boy, my impression of him had been largely shaped by how readily he would bring out the belt. In my young mind, that made him a formidable presence. It just no longer matched reality. The road accident had left him a shell of his former self. He had made progress in learning to walk with one stick, but without Noel he remained largely housebound. I'd arrive at his house to find him struggling to get out of his chair to greet me. As I shot up, making notable gains every time I saw him, Dad seemed to wither and age beyond his years. With that, his authority over me waned.

'I'll do it when I'm ready,' I snapped at him one time when he asked if I had completed my homework for the weekend. 'You can't order me about!'

Emotionally, our father had also become quite fragile. He no longer had the measured resolve that would leave us fearful of a summons to his study. Now, he was the one who shrank from anger, as if perhaps it would reveal just how vulnerable he'd become. It was completely understandable, given what he'd been through. Even so, for a period of time as I approached my sixteenth birthday I took advantage of that by finding issue with anything that sounded remotely like instruction. Admittedly, I was an adolescent who felt like his own mind and body had just been hotwired. I was angry at him, I suppose, and not just because I was beginning to question our parents' roles in our upbringing. The injuries he'd sustained in a car accident of his own making would leave him dependent on his children for the rest of his life. In the heat of any moment

I felt in his presence, it represented poor decisions that continued to have an impact on us all. I might well have directed the same feelings towards my mum had she been around. It's just once again she had completely removed herself from all responsibility. As our father couldn't escape any more, he became the focus for my frustrations.

Back at school, I began to regret those outbursts. It was the closest I came to behaving like those boys who abused their position to make our lives miserable. I felt bad about it, and yet at the time I couldn't bring myself to apologize. The feelings I'd been directing at Dad had been a long while in the making, and I still didn't fully understand them myself. All I knew for sure was that the balance of power had shifted towards his children and would never go back. He was too feeble now in mind and body. Our father's best days were behind him. Meanwhile, as I grew into myself, I began to see chinks of light opening up for me.

8

GIRLS AND CARS

Our sister school was situated just down the road from us. Less than a mile to the south, over 500 girls were educated just like us in a cluster of red-topped buildings amid generous grounds. For boys ranging in age from twelve to eighteen, this became a source of increasing fascination.

The two Potch schools had a close relationship with one another, and this included shared traditions. Every Sunday, in a formal and heavily scrutineered way, the boys would be permitted to visit the girls. One hour beforehand, the prefects gathered everyone outside the school in their role as chaperones. We would then walk down the road in an orderly fashion until we reached the gates of the other school.

There, we caught our first glimpse of the girls. They would be waiting outside the front of the main building, lined up side by side. Under instructions to conduct ourselves as gentlemen, we would file through the gates and then spread out wide to match their formation. Then, to the sound of more than 1,000 quickening heartbeats, and with everyone dressed in blazers and boaters, the boys would walk towards the girls. From above, it probably looked like two opposing armies squaring up for battle. Equipped with little more than hormones and flimsy introductions we'd rehearsed in the mirror, there could be no retreat. The two wide lines effectively matched a boy to a girl. Once face to face, we would greet our counterpart with a handshake. From there, we were permitted to break off and conduct a conversation with each other for a short time.

Even now, those weekly meets remain one of the most excruciatingly awkward experiences of my life.

The first time, facing a poor girl from the year above who was trying hard not to look disappointed, I thought I might self-combust with sheer embarrassment. I just didn't know what to say. Fortunately, my sister spotted me and swept in to save me from choking on my own name. Having inherited our mother's graceful looks, she also proved to be a popular draw. In her company, those boys who liked to pick on me suddenly became my best friends. Lindsay always saw through it, of course, and it was fun to watch her toying with them. Had she not stepped up to help me, I would have died on the spot. It was a huge relief when the boys were ordered to withdraw, and yet over time the encounter became a focal point for the week.

As my confidence continued to grow, so I began to enjoy the experience. At heart, I was quite a sociable boy, but after years of being knocked down and silenced my shell was still thicker than most. Among boys, I always worried that someone could turn on me without warning. That feeling went away during our weekly get-together with the opposite sex. It came with a significant risk of rejection, of course, but never ridicule. I liked meeting new people, even if I wasn't among those lucky few in later years who claimed their efforts had resulted in that most valuable of status symbols: a girlfriend.

Once a year, the two schools would stage a dance. This struck me as being a somewhat magical opportunity to meet the opposite sex. At the time, I was old enough to be very interested in girls but acutely aware of my shortcomings. Despite the weekly practice on the playing fields, I was still some gangly teenager who didn't feel like he was in full control of his limbs or the words that left his mouth. Nevertheless, I dressed up as smartly as I could for the evening, which was a challenge given I had no money to replace the clothes I'd outgrown, and told myself to make up for it by being charming and assertive.

If I was going to make an impression, I would need to step out of my comfort zone.

That evening, pressed to the wall of the hall along with all the other boys as the disco lights shimmered on the empty floor, I looked across at the girls on the other side and wondered how anyone got a romance off the ground. Eventually, some of the braver lads dared to cross the divide to ask for a dance. I just couldn't break free from my own self-doubts and insecurities. I had always been a nobody in school. Why would I expect girls to treat me any differently?

The only time I freely came out of my shell was on

stage. It was the last place I expected to find myself. I only joined the school's drama club because it seemed like a fun thing to do. It also took me away from the boarding house, and the chance of being in the wrong place at the wrong time. The club was run by the headmaster's wife, who had always been very kind to me. They'd put on a few productions, and I admired some of the boys I knew who had got involved. But with no girls in the club, since each school staged their own dramas, we had to improvise. As a result, my first role was as a female character who spent almost the entire production in the wings. I played a bride, beset by doubt, who had locked herself in the bathroom ahead of her wedding. My dialogue was minimal as I responded to those characters on stage trying to coax me out. In fact, I only joined them in the spotlight with my last line, as the bride is finally persuaded to unlock the door and join her fiancée. Wearing a wedding dress, and in striking makeup, I received a big laugh. I was part of a production that had a positive effect on people. It was a good feeling.

To celebrate, the headmaster's wife invited us all to the family house for tea and cake. The Ackermans lived on school grounds. It was a place I'd always considered to be out of bounds, and so I was a little wary about finding myself in the kitchen with the headmaster himself. Away from the school Mr Ackerman came across as a friendly guy who made every effort to make us boys feel at ease. They had four daughters, who joined us in the kitchen as the cake was cut and served. All of them were as striking as they were confident, especially the older two who were teenagers, and also quite relaxed around us.

Watching the pair interact with everyone, chatting to us and joking with their parents who were clearly so proud of them, it struck me that this was what a family should look like: a unit that could be stronger than the sum of its parts.

Over time, our visits to the Ackerman house for refreshments became a regular feature of drama club. As well as a place to celebrate putting on a production, we'd often be invited across after rehearsals. Each time, as I got to know the family, I felt more able to be myself. I enjoyed their company, but found myself drawn to one of the daughters in particular. Tracy was the same age as me. She attended the girls' school as a day pupil. Although I never managed to position myself in the right place in the line to meet her on a Saturday morning, we got along very well. I started to hope that she would be at home when we dropped in after drama club. Around the table, I'd dare to glance across at her. Sometimes, I'd find she was already looking at me. Eventually, I realized that I had feelings for her.

As a lovestruck sixteen-year-old high-school boy, the traditional way to ask someone out was by writing them a letter. On paper, this should have suited me. Frankly, the thought of doing so face to face left me unable to blink or breathe. At the same time, whenever I sat down with a pen in hand I found myself lost for words. I'd seen too many boys mooching around because their efforts had earned them a rejection. So, I bound up my affections inside my chest and hoped that one day Tracy would pick up on them.

Almost a year after joining the drama club, and becoming

a regular visitor to the house, I received an invitation that I couldn't turn down.

'Paul, we were wondering if you'd like to come on holiday with us?'

It was Mrs Ackerman who asked me – who by then had insisted I call her Ann – though Tracy was with her at the time and seemed to hold out for my answer. Over the course of twelve months, Ann had shown me such kindness that I had come to think of her as a kind of surrogate parent. She may well have known about my background, and also that we couldn't afford to go away in between terms. Whatever the case, I was bowled over by such a generous offer. Not least because it meant spending time with the girl I really liked.

The family had rented a beachside cottage just outside Durban: an east-coast city in the Natal province and a 400-mile drive from Potchefstroom. They had a big VW Combi with three rows of seats. With all the luggage packed, it was still a squeeze to fit in alongside the four daughters. I also had to get used to the fact that the man behind the wheel was off duty as a headmaster. In his shorts and sunglasses, and now quite clear that I should call him Hugo, this was just another dad looking forward to his holiday. Mr Ackerman could be quite authoritarian at school. Now, he seemed content to let the girls in his life call the shots, and that suited me just as much as him. Tracy and her sisters were witty and wise, and so generous in helping me to fit in. They also knew how to squabble, of course, which sometimes required their mother's intervention, but on the whole that long journey struck me as a bonding experience for the family. By the time we arrived, I felt like I belonged.

In the two weeks that followed, far removed from my life, I had never felt so happy. It was the first time that I could be myself without concern, and I had the Ackermans to thank for it. I joined in with chores, like cleaning and cooking, and enjoyed their company on walks, on the beach and splashing about in the water. Above all, of course, I had a chance to spend time with Tracy. We'd break off to hang out together, and sometimes even hold hands.

By the end of that first holiday, I was in the clutches of first love. Back at school, that was enough for me to sit down and write to ask Tracy if she would be my girlfriend. When she accepted my offer, I had visions of us walking into the sunset together. In reality, the school timetable and our exam year prevented us from seeing very much of each other. Even when we had time to ourselves, it was quite a chaste relationship. Tracy and I were young and finding our way as young adults. We both seemed content with the idea of being in a relationship rather than the reality. It was a happy time, and certainly enough for us both until we graduated from school and followed different paths in life. It also brought an unexpected reprieve from any further bullying. Inevitably, I suppose, dating the headmaster's daughter would earn that kind of amnesty. By the time it came to an end, I found that everyone had grown up while I'd gained some confidence to take care of myself.

9

ON INJUSTICE

I learned a great deal about myself during my time at Potchefstroom Boys High. I knew that my tendency to hold back on the edge of things was down to my early years, and that was fine. I learned to be comfortable with it, and frankly I wasn't alone in being a little reserved around people. That's where I found my tribe, in fact. We weren't the cool, brash kids, and nor did I want to be one. Having been picked on for so long, I was wary of anyone who sought attention at the expense of others.

Once the bullying trailed away, I considered myself to be a happy and reasonably outgoing kind of person. I also came to realize that I could be good at some things. The move to Potch had put paid to my plans to become a rower. I soon forgot about it, anyway, because the school offered a range of other sports that I enjoyed. Swimming was a strong point for me. I represented the school on several occasions and enjoyed feeling like I could be competitive. My late growth spurt worked in my favour in the water, but it was as a runner where my long legs and skinny frame really suited the demands of the sport. The athletics season soon became my favourite time to be outdoors. I loved time on the track. Sprinting wasn't my thing. It was just too frenetic and over as quickly as it began. What I loved to run were middle distances from 800 to 3,000 metres. There, I grew comfortable with pushing myself. I enjoyed the rivalry before the finish line, and the camaraderie on the other side. Above all, I liked how I felt at peace with myself afterwards.

By the time I approached my final year at the school, running felt like a pursuit that would stay with me in some shape or form.

In the classroom, I remained spectacularly average in everything but maths and science. So I decided that I should become a teacher in these subjects, which summed up my ambitions at the time. My life was defined by school, in and out of class. I just had no exposure to any other walk of life, and so a career in education seemed like the right step. After so much turmoil, I just wanted to enter my adult life feeling settled.

While I had a strong urge to put down roots, increasingly I found myself looking at the world around me and questioning my place in it. I had grown up in an English-speaking community in South Africa. We didn't have much to do with our white counterparts, the Afrikaners of Dutch heritage. I had to learn the language at school, but never got on with it. Nor could I see any reason to speak it. In my experience we pretty much existed independently from each other. It was a complex relationship largely dictated by the fact the ruling Afrikaners were the architects of apartheid. Established in 1948, this system of racial segregation and oppression towards the Black majority population was in full swing when I was born, and wasn't dismantled until the early nineties. Throughout my years in care and at school, the reality of what was happening in our country was carefully shaped and filtered by the authorities. Our news was heavily censored. Townships – those racially segregated and densely populated residential areas designated for Black residents – were out of sight and out of mind. In care and later at school, my only real exposure to that community came in the shape of housekeepers and gardeners. I was aware that they were seen as subservient roles. I just lived in a bubble that insulated us from the wider reality.

For me, that bubble was only pricked for the first time in the late seventies when a history teacher underwent a quiet crisis of faith in front of the class. In doing so, he opened my eyes to the shameful injustice of it all.

I remember the man as a very good storyteller. His lessons transported us to momentous events that shaped the world, and helped us to understand the significance. On this particular occasion, we had been covering South Africa's modern history. Our teacher stood at the front of the class with a textbook in hand, which he referenced from time to time to read out quotes from major figures who had shaped the country after the Second World War. As he read out a paragraph that presented those politicians who orchestrated apartheid as saviours of the nation, he halted mid-sentence. Closing the book, he drew breath, but then didn't seem to know what to say

'I . . . um . . . so . . .'

This sharpened my attention, as it did for every boy in the class. Our teacher was suddenly overwhelmed by some internal thought. He blinked rapidly, as if holding back tears, and then marched from the room so abruptly that we all looked at one another in astonishment.

A minute later, a boy by the window spotted him out on the step by a fire door. We watched him light up a cigarette, which he began to pull upon furiously. Nobody used the opportunity to fool about. We just sat there in an awkward silence until he returned to the classroom a few minutes later. Our teacher didn't say why he had taken off, but as he pressed on with the lesson I knew something momentous had just occurred. Something in that textbook hadn't sat right with him, and he didn't refer to it again. He looked relieved when the bell rang, as did most of my classmates who couldn't wait to tell everyone else about the meltdown we had witnessed. It was so out of character, and stayed with me for a long time.

That moment marked the start of a journey for me. It was a slow but steady awakening that many in my generation experienced. Talking to people proved to be an effective way of lifting the veil around us, especially those who were already wise to the reality of apartheid. It seemed to me that among the English community, people tolerated the situation even if they didn't agree with it, and yet their silence surely made them as complicit as those who believed it to be an entitlement. It was ugly, indefensible and to my young mind just deeply unfair. Activists who stood up to the establishment, like Nelson Mandela, were branded terrorists and imprisoned, while too many people living comfortable lives were unwilling to stand up and be counted.

The more I learned about our society and the entrenched belief that it couldn't be challenged, so my desire for my own independence grew stronger. I'd spent my entire life just following rules in an unfair system. If I was going to forge my own path, somehow I needed to feel qualified to do so. By the time I left school at seventeen I had a plan in place. First, I would go to university. A degree would open opportunities in teaching, which was really all I knew. So, I applied to study mathematics in Durban. I saw it as the first step on a flight into adulthood, and a chance to escape in some ways. It involved moving to a new city and taking responsibility for myself for the first time in my life.

Six months into my first year of study, after a reality check that hit me hard, I returned to Johannesburg.

My chosen degree had proven to be far tougher than I imagined. I had struggled from the start, and sensed myself falling behind with every week that passed. I dare say I might have recovered had I asked the university for help and support, but frankly I'd discovered that my heart just wasn't in the subject or even the prospect of teaching. I'd taken out a bank loan to support my living costs, and that rattled me. I didn't like being in debt. It felt like too much responsibility, and that just contributed to the feeling that I had made a mistake. Had I paused for breath, and reflected on why my confidence crumbled so quickly, I might have recognized that it was inevitable for someone with my background. I had grown up in institutional care, only to rush into the world so I could live my life. With no gradual transition, I had simply sunk.

Back home once again, I found my father had made slow but steady progress to recover some independence. He'd even moved out from my stepbrother's apartment into a small place nearby. Significantly, he had regained some sensation in the left-hand side of his body, which meant he was able to clean and cook for himself again as well as walk with a cane. While it was great to see he had made progress, I felt like my life had stalled.

With this in mind, it didn't take me long to regroup and work out where I should be. In my later years at high school, in fact, we'd all had to fill out official forms confirming our availability for two years' military service. Conscription was compulsory in South Africa. It meant at some point I would have to enrol. As a student, I could have deferred my service. That option was available to me if I stayed in education. My brother had done just that by signing up to an accountancy course. Even if I had decided to stay at university, I was well aware that at some point I'd have to put any career on hold to fulfil my service. Most people I knew got it out of the way at the earliest opportunity. As a dropout, having crashed and burned academically, I decided it might as well be now.

From an ideological point of view, joining a fighting force went against my newfound awareness of unfairness and injustice in South African society. I had no desire to contribute to the enforcement of apartheid. What's more, the country was in a state of tension at the time with neighbouring countries such as Mozambique, Angola and Namibia. With this in mind, and because of his service during the Second World War, my father recommended that I apply to the air force. He even called on his old contacts which made it all but a done deal. Without a doubt, I saw it as the soft option. Rather than risk finding myself on some kind of frontline, I would be more likely to be stationed at some obscure air base where I could quietly see out my duty. If I could thread an easy way through the twenty-four months that followed, I thought to myself, then perhaps this time back in the system would give me the chance to regroup and work out what I really wanted to do with my life.

While Dad had opened doors into the air force, I still had to undertake three months of basic training. During this time, the three forces would hand-pick those rookies who showed promise with a rifle. Concerned I might inadvertently possess some talent as a marksman, and find myself fast-tracked into action, I took steps to make sure I was hopeless. This just involved looking down the sights of a rifle as we were assessed on the range and finding the target belonging to the recruit next to me. That seemed to do the trick.

For those initial twelve weeks, I figured I had it all worked out. Other new recruits struggled with the transition from the comforts of home to military life. Many had never lived away from their parents. I was quite familiar with the discipline and the structured days. Where I encountered difficulties, I soon realized, was with those in command. Gone were the teachers with years of experience behind them. At the training camp, I found myself being ordered about by career officers whose seniority was no reflection of their intelligence.

Given that the army recruited from sixteen, some were also younger than me.

'Did you just tut, Sinton-Hewitt? That's twenty press-ups, right now!'

Within a short space of time, as I continued to bristle in the face of aggressive or unnecessary orders, I realized I had developed a problem with misplaced authority. After years of being too small or scared to stand up to it, now I found myself staring down my superiors if I felt they were trying to score points.

Inevitably, it only invited more trouble.

Before our three-month induction was over, I earned myself a string of punishments. The worst involved running repeatedly up and down a hill carrying two car tyres. I'd provoked the young officer into making an example of me by refusing to have my tunic dry-cleaned over several weeks. In my view, he had only instructed me to do it so he could throw his weight about. It wasn't dirty, and I had no intention of submitting. Now I found myself on a steep slope, red dirt underfoot, a fiery sun overhead and an audience on both sides of recruits who had stepped out of their billets to watch me. The officer insisted that I press on until I dropped, and I was determined to stay on my feet. We were being as stubborn and belligerent as each other, but I wasn't calling the shots. After hours of hill repeats carrying a heavy load, having been sick down my fatigues, he finally ordered me to stand down. I collapsed on the spot, and had to be carried back to my quarters.

'Just be ready for inspection first thing tomorrow morning,' he growled, as my bunkmates hauled me over the threshold.

The tunic I had to present was sodden with sweat, dirt and puke. I was also beyond exhaustion, which is where my fellow recruits stepped in to help me. They dumped me in the shower, where I lay motionless for half an hour under the streaming water. When I finally came to my senses, I found they had washed my uniform. I had to stay up late, repeatedly ironing every item until it was all dry, and then next day the inspection passed without incident.

As far as the officer was concerned, he had broken me. In my mind, I had won by not giving in, but above all the experience had taught me more about the power of collective kindness. My billet mates had come together to save me from further punishment, for which I thanked them all. While I questioned if my attitude to authority was a strength or a weakness, I just hoped that in their boots I would have also reserved judgement and done the right thing.

By the end of our training period, I was ready for the air force. Some of my fellow graduates saw my posting to a sleepy outpost miles from anywhere as some kind of failure. I was more than happy with that outcome. There, I would be trained in interpreting aerial activity by radar, and that suited me down to the ground. I spent much of the time deep in an underground bunker, monitoring planes at my workstation, working out height and trajectory, and calling out positions. I found it really interesting on a technical level. It all came down to process. After years of following rules, it felt quite natural to me and also refreshing to be in a role where I could eventually suggest refinements. After some time, I even served as the instructor for a new intake of recruits. I enjoyed breaking down the tasks involved so others could learn. I even had authority over them, much like the officer I had squared up to in training. On being promoted to the next rung on the ladder, my role as their corporal extended to leading marching practice and daily billet inspections. I never felt the need to overstep the mark in the same way as the officer who had tangled with me in training, though goodness knows what those young conscripts made of me. By then, fairness had become the touchstone in my life. I was nineteen years old, living in an unjust society, and it informed everything I did.

10

THE WORLD AROUND

To my surprise, I was quite sad to serve my final day at the air base. Over the course of two years I had made good friends, developed a genuine interest in how systems worked, and not once fired a gun in anger. To my mind, that was mission accomplished. According to the rules of conscription, I was still required to return to uniform for several months over the course of the next ten years, but in effect the bulk of my military service was done.

As the end approached, I was mindful that once again I would be leaving institutional life. Having tripped over myself in my first taste of independence as a university student, I didn't want to make the same mistake again.

So, rather than rushing into finding work, I decided to broaden my horizons. Throughout my service, I had continued to switch on to the way society worked. That conscription in the seventies only applied to white South

Africans was just another example of how apartheid dictated every aspect of our lives. It empowered people like me while impoverishing others based solely on the colour of their skin. My generation had been born into it, though many were challenging the sense of resignation that allowed the system to perpetuate. As well as instilling in me a rising distaste for authority, it encouraged my view that there must be more to the world. When I returned to Johannesburg, my father made a suggestion that seemed like exactly the right thing to do at that moment in time.

'Why don't you visit Scotland?' said the man who had left the country behind for a life in South Africa. 'You have family there, after all.'

Family. That word had always resonated with me. Mostly because I knew that my understanding of it was different from everyone else. I had never considered that mine was bigger than the broken remains that we'd lived with since going into care. Now I had an opportunity to explore it on a wider level. To his credit, Dad shared my excitement. Despite the diligent work he put into regaining his mobility and independence, his accident had left him in a world that was smaller than before. As a result, he had developed an appreciation for the simple but more meaningful things in life. His drive for social status was all but gone, and in its place a genuine sense of enthusiasm that his youngest son was set to explore his roots.

It was my father who volunteered to contact relatives who still lived in Newtongrange, the coal-mining village outside Edinburgh where he had been raised. His mother still lived there, but she was very old and in care. With help from his various distant cousins, Dad put arrangements into place while I planned to extend my adventures with a whistlestop tour of Europe. Having never travelled before, my understanding of what lay beyond our borders came down to what I had learned at school, and from movies and the news.

Within a short space of time, arrangements had been made and I was at the airport saying goodbye to Noel and my father. Timmy had also joined us, having moved in with Dad while he studied accountancy. The day before I'd called my sister to say goodbye. She seemed so much older than me now, and more settled in her life with work and a partner. While I felt more prepared to face the world than I had when I set off for university, I was still nervous about the trip. I had never been on a plane before. In fact, I hadn't left the country since my arrival as a newborn when Dad brought my mother and me back from Rhodesia. Shortly after my birth, he had added me to his passport. As my father was a native Australian, and I needed my own passport to travel, that entitled me to apply for one from the Australian High Commission. It all happened very quickly, but reinforced my desire to get away from South Africa and its segregated society.

'I'll bring you a gift,' I said to Timmy, on hoisting my rucksack onto my back, because I knew he'd only ask. 'Something you'd least expect!'

It felt very strange turning away from them all and heading for the gates. Through glass partition walls, every time I looked around, I could see them watching me. A customs officer in a kiosk had just finished processing a passenger's documentation in front of me. I waved one final time at Dad, Timmy and Noel and then placed my new Australian passport on the counter.

The officer flicked through the blank, box-fresh pages, and then carefully considered me.

'One-way trip?' he asked.

'Back in six weeks,' I said brightly, only for him to slide the passport back to me.

'Only nationals have a right to return,' said the officer, and then tapped on the Australian coat of arms embossed on the cover. 'Where's your authorized permission?'

His response left me momentarily lost for words. I'd lived in South Africa for all but the first few months of my life. I'd also recently completed military service, I told him when I finally found my voice, but the guy had only one response.

'You're free to leave, but as a visitor you'll need paperwork to come back.'

'One moment.'

I turned to the glass partition. On the other side, my father and Noel had seen something was wrong. They couldn't hear a word I said as I tried to relay the problem. In that moment, it felt like I was in some kind of no man's land. Not only was I feeling increasingly disillusioned by the country I was leaving, but it also seemed the country had no place for me anyway. Eventually, after several attempts, my stepbrother understood what had happened. He conferred with our father for a moment. Dad nodded, looking concerned, and then grinned at me.

'*Go!*' he mouthed, waving me on with his stick, before conveying that he would address the situation while I was away.

Knowing the efforts he would go on to make to secure

the documentation I needed, this was the moment my father finally stepped up for me unconditionally. When he passed away, just a few years later, I would remember him as a man who overcame so many challenges in life to find his true self.

The journey to Scotland was an adventure in its own right. It seemed like almost everyone on board my flight to Heathrow was a smoker, which was permitted on planes at the time. When I disembarked, the smell of cigarettes was in my hair and clothes, and followed me into London where I stayed overnight at a cheap boarding house. The capital completely overwhelmed me. The sheer scale of everything was like nothing I had seen before, from the buildings to the crowds and the traffic. As for the tube system, I saw people flocking into entrances to the Underground and rising out of exits and decided it was far too complicated for me. Having walked to the coach station with the rucksack on my back, I couldn't wait to be on the long ride to Edinburgh. By the time I arrived at the address I had been given in the town just outside the city, I was tired and hungry, in need of a wash and disorientated by jetlag. One of my father's cousins had offered to host me. I knew her name was Betty, and that was it.

I was also aware that quite a few members of this extended family lived in and around Newtongrange. I just hadn't anticipated that they would all have come out to greet me. As I paused to smarten myself up before knocking, the front door opened. A broad, rosy-faced woman in her finery beamed at me, before a whole host of people spilled out around her as if this was the highlight of their day. All of them had dressed up. They looked like they had just returned from a church service.

'Paul!' she declared, having introduced herself as my host. 'How lovely to meet you!'

At once, I was pulled into a string of hugs and handshakes by Betty and relatives whose existence I knew virtually nothing about. I knew most of the names but not the faces, and yet every single one was warm, welcoming and friendly. I also realized they had made the effort for me. I felt quite overwhelmed. Nobody in my family had shown me this degree of enthusiasm in my whole life.

And it had only just begun.

Inside, I was escorted into the front room for tea and cake. Betty had also laid out photograph albums of old pictures of my father as a boy. As she took me through each page, she pointed out people in the room who appeared in some of the shots as younger versions of themselves. It felt like a living history, and I loved every moment. Betty even went on to open a bottle of South African wine that my father had shipped back when he first emigrated.

'For a special occasion,' she said, uncorking the bottle with some ceremony.

At once, the smell of vinegar filled the air. One sip told me it had gone off years ago, and I can only think everyone was too polite to point it out. Still, with all the toasts I managed to finish my glass. It was such a wonderful reception. People were talking to me from all directions, and in an accent I sometimes found hard to follow, but their intent was clear. I was a welcome guest in this house. We were family, after all.

I stayed with Betty for a fortnight. In that time, various relatives took me on excursions and tours. I walked the hills outside Edinburgh and visited the castle where my father's famous photograph of the downed bomber was on display. Betty even took me to visit my grandmother. It was a bittersweet encounter, for she was in the grip of dementia and failed to register either of us. Still, I was so grateful to Betty because she knew how much it meant to me. I experienced such generous hospitality throughout, and yet it was one exchange outside my Scottish family circle that came to define my stay.

'Who do you think you are?'

'I'm sorry?'

The question came from one of my cousin's friends; a young man about my age who played tennis. Betty had suggested that he take me to the local court for a game, which seemed like a good idea at the time. It had started pleasantly enough, with gentle serves from my opponent as he gauged my ability. Shortly into the session though, I sensed he seemed tense for some reason. Then, when I caught his eye, it wasn't just a sharp serve that caught me off guard.

'You've got a nerve,' he said next, as I collected the ball. 'A racist like you coming here.'

I stopped in my tracks and faced him again.

'I'm not a racist,' I said, which prompted an incredulous laugh.

'Paul, you're a white South African. The way you treat the Black population is disgusting! You should be ashamed of yourself.'

I felt my face turning hot in shock as much as embarrassment. His anger was clear, not just in his accusation but the force with which he served the next ball right at me. It caught me on the leg and stung.

'I'm not South African,' I said, mostly to myself in that moment, for I had no other response for him.

The incident haunted me. I didn't like the apartheid system one bit, but I had never considered that I should be held responsible. I had no idea that people outside the country viewed us with such animosity. I had always viewed the system as something that was imposed on us. Now it felt as if I was complicit in its existence. From that moment on, free from the media restrictions back home, I began to learn the unvarnished truth. I'd never heard of the Soweto Uprising or the Sharpeville Massacre: two anti-apartheid protests quelled by a brutal police force that had caused outrage outside South Africa. Here in the UK, the African National Congress Party weren't considered a terrorist organization – as presented to the people of South Africa by the authorities – but a force for freedom from oppression. I knew about the economic sanctions imposed upon our country, but they had always been sold to us as attacks on our sovereignty by foreign powers to further their own interests. What was entirely new to me was that the entire world seemed united in its condemnation of our government. Protests and marches were a regular feature of life across Europe and other continents. People had strong opinions here. They knew right from wrong.

I was ashamed by what I learned, and also angry that a state could use censorship and propaganda to impose their will and then leave its citizens feeling responsible. It certainly wasn't something I felt comfortable talking about to Betty and my relatives. I was at the end of my stay in Scotland and needed time to process it.

Over the course of the next month, having said goodbye to the Newtongrange clan, I journeyed by bus from London to Paris, Amsterdam and Venice. It took me a while to acclimatize to each new city. It was as if my senses were heightened as I explored and took in the sights. I registered every detail, but what struck me most was how the world outside my homeland was completely multicultural. There was an equality here, and it made each place richer for it. I was old enough to know it wasn't perfect, but a harmony existed that I had never experienced. If anything, it furthered my sense of detachment from the place I called home. I felt no particular loyalty to South Africa. When I called my dad from a phone box, I should have been relieved when he told me that I had permission to return. I just had to visit the High Commission in London to collect the documentation. I realized he had gone to great lengths for me to sort it out. I had also seen how important family could be. Even though I felt quite flat about the prospect, I had a duty to go back.

My trip had certainly opened my eyes. What I learned came as a surprise, but I also felt more comfortable now I knew the truth. I had set out to widen my experience of life and that helped me to understand my place in it. Six weeks later, I returned to South Africa with a heightened disdain for authority and a sense that the state could no longer control how I chose to live my life.

11

THE GREAT ESCAPE

The package arrived just over a month after my return. I had posted it to myself from London. I thought the surprise I had promised my brother would amuse him. I also considered it to be a small act of defiance against the authorities, because in South Africa the content was banned.

There had been many things that were new and surprising to me in the UK. Adult magazines were a case in point. In South Africa, the top shelf in the newsagent wasn't reserved for soft pornography, as it was banned on grounds of immorality. So, with my brother in mind, but also still rankled by what the country now represented to me, I decided to buy two magazines and post them home.

It hadn't occurred to me that the South African authorities would have the right or inclination to monitor and intercept the mail of a twenty-year-old backpacker on a European adventure, and even then deem it worthy of action. When I opened the package, I didn't even notice the parcel tape along the seal that wasn't there when I sent it.

'Hey, Timmy, I've got something for you!

My brother worked hard, but also liked to make the most of his free time. He had an exciting social life compared to mine, and I hoped it would make him think I could be fun to be around. At first, Timmy was taken aback by what I had presented him. Then a goofy grin spread across his face, as I had hoped. But it didn't last long.

'Isn't this illegal?' he said, and though he laughed on leafing quickly through the pages, it left me feeling like the reality of my surprise didn't match my expectation.

I felt a little foolish when he handed it back. Soon afterwards, I decided that the best place for the magazines would be in the bin.

A few days later, I answered a knock at the door.

'Can I help?' I asked, surprised to find four policemen on the doorstep.

'We're here to arrest you,' said one, and told me I'd know why.

Despite feeling like my heart had momentarily stopped beating, I feigned ignorance. Even as the leading officer spelled out their reasons for arresting me, I maintained a puzzled expression and shook my head.

'There are no magazines here,' I said, which was the truth, as I knew the refuse truck had done the rounds the morning before.

The officer responded by asking me to stand aside while they searched the premises.

Luckily, I was alone in the house when the raid took

place. All I could do was continue to look bewildered as the police turned the place upside down. It was a deeply unpleasant experience, and lasted almost an hour. From the moment I had opened the door to the raid, I realized my mail must have been intercepted. I was also aware that they knew full well contraband material had arrived at this address. I just didn't know what would happen next. We had all heard stories about how corrupt the police could be. As the police continued their search, it felt like my whole life had suddenly come adrift. It was out of my control, and in the hands of a force I couldn't trust. So, when the officer in charge called off the search and instructed his men to exit the premises, I was braced to be told that unless I paid him off he would say that they had found something.

Instead, the officer paused at the door to glower at me.

'There's nothing here,' he said, as if every word pained him. 'But I'm watching you now.'

It would be the last time I ever saw the man, but I'd learned my lesson. Smuggling in those magazines had been a reckless thing to do. It also brought home the fact that the South African state had the capacity to ruin lives. I had been an idiot at a time when I was preparing to spread my wings. From that moment on, as if defaulting to the boy just trying to survive, it focused me on doing what I saw as the right thing. I needed to find work rather than follow any wanderlust, build a career and settle down. With those foundations, I decided, the future would eventually be mine to determine.

It was the early eighties. The computer revolution was in full swing and stock markets were set to go boom. As a young man with an interest in systems, and a stepbrother who had found success working on the frontier of computer technology, I saw a path that I could follow.

With my new suit and tie, I began working as a trainee junior programmer for one of the big financial houses in Johannesburg. Noel had described the machines he worked with as being quite bulky. I hadn't anticipated that at the time a single computer occupied an entire room. I was assigned to one that bristled with lights and switches, hummed like the engine room of a liner and produced enough heat for my shirt to stick to my skin. In those days, programming a computer wasn't a question of writing complicated code. It literally came down to punching holes in cards that would be fed into the computer to execute a command. Learning the sequences was painstaking and laborious, but it all came down to procedures.

Having been raised in a system, and then found an aptitude for working within them as an instructor at the air base, it all felt quite intuitive. I had to knuckle down to learn the new technology and create programmes from scratch that helped the bank move towards a more automated approach. Even though I was only on the first rung of the ladder, it felt like the makings of a career.

'Where would you like to be in five years from now?' asked the woman from HR who was tasked with my first appraisal.

It was a question I hadn't seriously considered before, not just in this job but in my life more broadly. It was difficult to answer in any detail. With no real guidance in my life, I just tended to think in terms that were both wildly ambitious and idealistic.

'Well,' I finally answered in a bid to at least sound confident and knowledgeable, 'I'd like to be the general manager.'

As a young trainee programmer with no actual banking skills, I might as well have declared that I'd be running for president. The HR woman nodded, seemingly satisfied, and quietly jotted something next to the question on her clipboard. I sat across from her thinking it was all going very well.

Despite coming across as a bit of a dreamer, I was good at my job. There was no way that I would be heading up the bank, but within a year I'd joined a small team within the vast organization that worked on delivering the country's first automated cash machine. With a regular wage, I was beginning to enjoy some stability. I was still living with my brother and my dad, but the financial independence was welcome. The next step, in my mind, was to move out and decide what I wanted to do with my life on my own terms. My first few attempts hadn't been easy. Now, I felt I had the maturity and experience to thrive.

Only one thing stood in my way. It was spelled out to me in a letter I received. I had also known it was coming. Having completed my mandatory two years of military service, I was obligated to return to camp for a month or so every two years for the next decade. It was a huge undertaking, but one that applied nationwide to every conscript. Essentially, it was just a part of life in South Africa. Companies made provisions for it, as did those who found themselves back at camp in military fatigues. By now, though, my ties to the country felt increasingly flimsy. I felt nothing but frustration at having to put my career on hold to serve the state. The last thing I wanted to do was return to scanning radars and living the regimented life I'd worked so hard to put behind me.

I stewed on the contents of the letter for a few days. Then, as it stirred up all the patriotic misgivings that had taken shape on my European tour, I decided to write to the authorities. The difficulties I'd had in just getting back into South Africa made me think that perhaps I could argue for exemption. *As a Southern Rhodesian by birth and an Australian passport holder*, I began, *surely it's not right that I should be asked to serve?* I pointed out that I had already completed the main bulk of my conscription but now wished to exercise the right to withdraw from further call-ups. It felt like a long shot, and I was braced for it to be dismissed.

I didn't even receive a reply. Every day I'd check the mail, but it became quite clear to me that my little objection had come to nothing. The system was just too big to listen to little people like me. I had no choice. As a natural-born South African, my brother had yet to answer the call-up. He constantly deferred by putting education and work first. Having already signed up to the process, I resigned myself to the fact that over the course of the next decade I would have to fulfil my duty to the state.

For a couple of months every two years, I returned to my role as a radar operator. I was posted to different camps across the country, which at least made things marginally more interesting. Even so, there was little to distract me from feeling like one of the punched holes in the cards I constructed; there to fulfil a task, when I could be at work creating the whole programme.

On a month-long posting in my third year, just as I had

resigned myself to the fact that my life would be interrupted in this way until I turned thirty, everything changed.

It happened quite by chance, following a brief exchange with another conscript I was friendly with as we passed one another outside the barracks.

'I've just been looking at my record in the sergeant major's office,' he told me. 'It's really interesting.'

'You can do that?'

'Sure!' he said, as if it was common knowledge. 'Everyone has a right to see their files.'

I had been on my way to the radar bunker to pull another shift. With a little time in hand, and out of sheer curiosity, I decided to make a detour.

On hearing my request, the sergeant major looked at me like it was the last thing he needed. It was indeed a right, he confirmed, but also a waste of his hard-pressed time. The last thing he wanted, he added, was for word to spread and bring a string of conscripts to his desk. Nonetheless, he crossed to a filing cabinet and began to rifle through the files. From where I was standing, they all looked very thin. I guessed each soldier had an identity record and little else.

Then he paused to wrestle out a file that had to be two inches thick.

'Sinton-Hewitt?' he said, having checked my surname matched the one stamped on the front, and then turned to hand it to me. 'What do we have on you, eh?'

Just then, I knew that if I sat down to read the contents of this hefty file I would be late for my shift. I also knew that opening it up was more important than any punishment. What I read took my breath away. Having flicked through the pages, I pulled out a sheet when I recognized my own handwriting. It was the letter I had penned as an Australian passport holder asking to be relieved from further duty. It was stamped to acknowledge receipt, some three years earlier, with documents clipped underneath it that confirmed I did indeed have a case. Only I had never been notified.

Despite his initial irritation at my request, the sergeant major had always been quite a reasonable chap. I placed the stamped letter in front of him on returning to his desk, along with the response from the higher-ups. Then I watched him turn red in the face as he worked through it all. The poor guy was in a bind. Here I was, an Australian in the pay of the South African Defence Force, with documentation to prove it should never have been allowed to happen. I was exempt. Had I known, I could have avoided conscription completely. Worse for them, when I had made the point they had buried it. The military machine had ground on.

'Come with me,' he said eventually, closing the dossier and rising from his desk.

As we crossed from the administrative building to my barracks, I could only think that immediate responsibility for the situation fell to him as the senior ranking officer at the base. Whether or not it had been on him to read my files in the first place, he looked as shocked as I felt. I didn't question him when he asked me to collect my belongings. A few minutes later, with everything packed into my kit bag, he led me to the main gates of the air base.

'So, I'm done?' I asked.

The sergeant major took a step back to salute, and then turned on his heels.

People said that I would have a case in court, but I didn't have any interest in pursuing it. Having been marched off the premises, and effectively discharged from further duty, it felt like I had scored a victory. With no further call-ups to get in the way of work, I could focus on building my career. I was also saving to buy a plot of land just outside Johannesburg so that I could build a house of my own. All that was missing from my life was someone to share it with.

This urge to do what society expected of me, fostered in a care system from an early age, was at odds with my disdain for the state. A quiet voice inside me wanted to cut loose from South Africa and start afresh, but a louder voice set out a more conventional path before I could possibly think about making that decision for myself.

The police raid, coupled with the military service debacle, had left me reverting to that ingrained instinct I had to comply for the sake of a quiet existence.

If anything, such a conflict in my mind should have warned me to pause and seek some clarity about what I really wanted from life. I needed to make informed decisions, and that would take time. Instead, one afternoon at the local swimming pool, I found myself drawn to a striking young woman reading a book in the sunshine. She had registered me and smiled back. Just then, bewitched by the attention, I knew that I had to find the courage to start a conversation. Even if I wasn't truly ready for the commitment that followed.

PART TWO

Bushy Park, Richmond, south-west London
Saturday, 4 October 2004
8.57 a.m.

'Welcome, everybody, and thank you for joining me here.'

I have no need to raise my voice to be heard by the small band of runners on the start line. Eight men and five women have assembled behind the edge of the yellow box junction on one side of the car park. They wear a mixture of club vests and casual t-shirts, athletics shorts and leggings. I know most of them, and really appreciate their support, but I'm thrilled to see several unfamiliar faces too. Even better, before I started my briefing of sorts, the group were chatting freely with one another.

This is what it's all about, I had thought to myself, and then gathered everyone to address them.

'If you lose your way, don't worry,' I say now, having described what is an unmarked but intuitive course shaped by paths and trees. It will take the runners on a 5K loop around the

perimeter that finishes close to where we're gathered, just off the car park beside a stream. There, a parade of trees set back from the water's edge forms a natural funnel I intend to use as the finish. It's a light touch in line with my aim for us all to be in and out of the park with minimal disruption to other users. I just hope that whoever leads the way has studied the course map I provided on the flyer. 'You can always have another go next week,' I add, just in case. 'I'll be here. Same time. Same place. So, you'll have to come back anyway if you want to try beating your time.'

Despite the ripple of laughter, most runners don't look like they can think beyond the 5K ahead of them. Some prime their watches, ready to time themselves. Others jump up and down on the spot or shift their weight from side to side. A few just smile at me, arms folded against a slight chill, ready to be on their way.

It's time. At last.

First checking that the opening stretch of the course is clear, I step back onto the double yellow lines at the edge of the car park. In response, some of the runners brace themselves to burst into action. Others stand there looking quite relaxed, which is absolutely fine by me.

'Take care of each other,' I say as my final piece of advice, feeling a mixture of excitement and nerves, but mostly just happiness at being in good company. 'Three, two, one . . .'

12

LIFELINES

By the mid-nineties, my career was flying high. After just over a decade working with software systems, I had climbed from being a junior programmer to a technical specialist. As one opportunity after the next opened up before me, I found myself operating internationally. That meant putting South Africa behind me for posts in Belgium, Denmark and ultimately the UK. England was my home now. I even had a British passport, thanks to my father's side of the family.

On paper, I was going places.

Professionally, I was responsible for big budgets, large numbers of personnel and delivering projects to deadline. Over time, I had risen to become one of those international frequent flyers, as well as a familiar face to head-hunters tasked with appointing someone capable of managing ventures with a level head and logical mind. My reputation in the industry was shorthand for success, and I had worked hard to achieve that.

On a personal level, I had crashed and burned. Internally, I was in pieces.

Since meeting the young woman at a swimming pool over ten years earlier, who I would go on to marry soon after, there followed the slow, painful realization that I wasn't ready for this stage in life. I had raced into a relationship and settled down because that seemed like the right thing to do. I acted with the best of intentions, of course, and the sense of happiness and stability it created felt like a refuge to someone with my turbulent background. Through my eyes, I was following a process into the wider world. From a young age, that was how I had believed life should be. Emerging from an institutional existence, I had no idea that people needed to truly find themselves before they could commit to anyone else. My marriage might have felt like a safe place, but no relationship can thrive without solid foundations.

By the time we relocated to Europe, following work opportunities on the mainland before gravitating to the UK, my wife and I were parents to two beautiful children. While raising our daughter and son, we were also experiencing growing difficulties as a couple. While I continued to tread a path that was expected of me, at home and in work, I also knew that I couldn't hold the system in which I'd been raised accountable for every move I made along the way. Yes, I had grown up to follow rules and conventions or face consequences. This mindset had been central to my childhood. It's what led me to think that if I didn't settle down and start a family as convention dictated then

I would be seen as a failure. As an adult, however, I still had to take responsibility for my feelings and decisions as our marriage teetered and then collapsed. The breakdown, separation and divorce was traumatic for us all. It caused lasting fault lines through our relationships and left me living alone in Twickenham, south-west London. I was devastated and in need of help.

'Should we start with the divorce?'

Sitting across from me, the personal counsellor considered my suggestion. I had come to her because I believed that I was broken. I had just turned thirty-five. My life was in turmoil. I was navigating fatherhood from afar while work had taken me in a direction that kept piling on more travel and responsibilities. As much as I told myself that my career was the one constant in my life that kept me grounded, it also brought a great deal of pressure and stress. I was also struggling to rebuild my life as a single man. I'd been on a few dates, but this is where a pattern had formed that troubled me. I couldn't seem to make anything last. Just as it felt as if I had met someone I liked, I'd peer into the future and panic. The way I saw myself, scarred by the collapse of my marriage, I wasn't equipped to sustain a relationship. I'd end up calling a halt to things without any clear reason, often out of the blue, which caused upset and left me feeling hollow and unhappy.

At a low point following yet another sour ending, and feeling both fragile and overwhelmed by life in general, I checked in with my doctor. In a lost and lonely place, I had found myself occupied by darkening thoughts. In those moments, I felt like I didn't want to be here any more. When I shared this with my GP, trying hard to underplay it while asking myself if I was just wasting his time, the doctor recommended that I seek counselling.

I was sceptical at first. Opening up about my thoughts and feelings didn't feel like a comfortable prospect for a quiet, reserved person like me. All I knew for certain was that I could no longer manage on my own. When I found the courage to take up the referral, I assumed the counsellor I met would want to explore what I considered to be the most significant relationship breakdown in my life. The end of my marriage had left me feeling like I was just presenting a functioning version of myself. At work, in a busy, pressured environment, I could switch off from everything but the task at hand. At the end of each day, however, I would be back at home or in a hotel room and at the mercy of suicidal thoughts. There was no escape from the sorrow, guilt, anguish and despair, and steadily the need to contain those feelings had exhausted me.

When I suggested beginning there, after the counsellor had encouraged me to introduce myself through the waypoints of my life, she asked me to go back even further.

'Let's talk about your mother,' she said, to my surprise. 'Tell me what she means to you.'

It was the last thing I expected to discuss. After all, she was referring to a figure who had remained distant from me throughout my adult years. Mum had made very little effort to reach out, but then nor had I. After Dad had died, it felt to me as if she no longer had much bearing on my life at all. Her relationship with the estate agent had ended and she subsequently met and married a new man called Ian. Together, they had moved to a small house by the beach in Natal Province with two dogs and less of the decadence that had once defined her.

As a family, it had seemed to me that we'd all moved on.

My sister lived in the same province as our mother, with a husband and children of her own. Lindsay and I were on good terms but somewhat distant. The disconnect that existed between us at school had only widened. Having shared so much of our institutional upbringing, my brother and I had more in common. Like me, Tim – as we now called him – had moved to England. He had worked hard on building a successful accountancy business, and was broadening his professional horizons as an entrepreneur. Tim was a busy man, but we still saw each other on occasion. When we did so, and our mother came up in conversation, he took a hardline view. *What did she do for us?* Tim would say. *Forget about her.*

While I didn't cut her out completely, as he had done as an act of self-preservation, my telephone calls were few and far between. Over the years, despite starting another relationship that outwardly seemed to bring her some contentment, Mum's drinking had escalated. Whenever we had dropped in on her from The Sons of England Care Home, she would always have a glass of wine on the go. Now, it seemed, that habit had crept insidiously towards alcohol addiction. She was very good at functioning, presenting herself as sharp and attuned. Even so, I could tell straight away when I called because she just didn't listen. Instead, she talked about herself with no apparent awareness, frequently repeating stories. It reached a point where I knew that if I wanted just a scrap of rewarding conversation I'd need to catch her first thing in the morning. Then, I could speak to my mother and feel that I wasn't wasting my breath. Beyond midday, when it felt like she was consciously trying not to slur her words, it was just upsetting.

Now, I found myself facing a counsellor who was encouraging me to open up about every aspect of my relationship with her. Anxious to please, despite failing to see how my mother could have any bearing on the way I was feeling, I did my best to answer her questions. Then, as I began to find my way into the subject, the therapist's prompts fell away and I just talked and talked.

Over the course of the sessions that followed, my mother was at the heart of everything we explored. It came with emotion, too, as I gradually came to understand the consequences of her decision to walk out on her children. I was a little boy when she left, and yet that abandonment continued to have a bearing on my life. In the hands of the therapist, the steady reveal cast a light on my past from a different perspective. Suddenly, things made sense. For much of my life, I had carried around some misplaced feeling of responsibility; that somehow I had not been enough for her. By extension, that had seeped into my outlook on relationships and effectively undermined them.

As well as the impact on my self-worth, I realized my mother's actions had also shaped my coping mechanisms. Admitting I needed help was out of character for me, the therapist suggested. I had only done so because I felt I'd reached rock bottom, but she was right. Having grown up with nobody to listen to my worries or step in to sort things out, I had become a closed book. Over the years I'd developed internal strategies to cope with whatever life threw at me. When faced with a problem, I'd set out to resolve it myself, rather than involving others with a stake in it or who could provide insight and contribute to solutions. This introspective and even stubbornly resolute approach wasn't constructive in my marriage and the failed relationships that followed. I might have got away with it at work but it wasn't good for my mental wellbeing. Ultimately, it had led me to the brink. In short, I needed to be more open about what was going on inside my mind, and not just shut people out.

After twelve challenging weeks of counselling, I felt as though I had begun to make peace with my past. At the start, I'd had no idea the sense of despair that led me there was just a symptom of a more deep-seated cause. With some clarity at last, I felt better equipped to deal with life. It didn't change my circumstances, but at least now I had a better understanding of myself. In a way, I had become my own project and that gave me order and shape to what I was facing. I also recognized I was prone to feelings that bordered on depression and would sometimes sink into it. The counsellor and I spent time talking about coping strategies. I had come to appreciate that talking was an effective way to make sense of what was spinning around inside my head. After all, that was what I had experienced over these three intense months, and which had effectively saved my life. While I didn't have many close friends in England who I could easily confide in, mostly because I moved around so much with work, I was determined that should change.

As the last session came to an end, the therapist suggested another way I could be kinder to myself. The subject came up a few times during our chats because it had already crept into my world long before leaving South Africa. Until this moment, however, I hadn't considered my love of running could help me to escape the hole in which I found myself. Generally, I saw it as an activity that helped me to stay fit. It provided me with goals that were exclusively based on pace and times. I was aware that I looked forward to lacing up my trainers. I also liked the feeling afterwards from the physical exertion. What I hadn't done was make the conscious connection between running and mental wellbeing.

'It gives you time out from everyday life,' said the counsellor to expand on this, before closing the notebook on her lap, 'and brings you together with other people.'

13

ON RUNNING

At school, it was an activity that gave me a sense of freedom. From the primary school playing field to the high school track, putting one foot in front of the other was something I enjoyed. It also helped me to feel like an equal, rather than the kid who held himself back from others.

In South Africa, running also carried cultural importance. During apartheid, when the country was banned from taking part in international occasions, such as the Olympics and the World Cup, our televised sporting calendar focused on domestic events. Central to this, alongside cricket and rugby, was an annual road race between the cities of Durban and Pietermaritzburg. The 88K race had been staged annually since 1921. It also played an instrumental role in breaking down apartheid policies by becoming racially integrated from 1975. The race still takes place to this day and is known as the world's oldest and largest ultramarathon.

When I first tuned in to watch the race at high school, in the year that our boarding house first got a television, coverage didn't just begin with the firing of the start gun. Programming spanned the entire day. It was a cause for national unity, which was a rare thing. The sheer scale was breathtaking. Thousands of runners took part, with eleven hours available to reach the finish. They seemed to flow as one along streets that were flanked the entire length of the course by cheering crowds. I loved the build-up and the excitement before the start, and just marvelled at the grit shown by all participants to run a distance that made my head spin.

Like so many people, I chose to watch the Comrades Marathon from the comfort of a sofa. My interest stayed with me long after high school. Into the eighties, I marvelled at the achievement of an incredible young runner and staunch anti-apartheid campaigner. Instantly recognisable by his long blonde hair and metronomic pacing, Bruce Fordyce would go on to win the event on a record nine occasions. As a runner, he became a national treasure. Long before running took over my life, the man was an inspiration to me.

In countries like the UK and USA, running solo – or jogging as it was more commonly known at the time – was considered to be somewhat niche. In South Africa, where Comrades had popularized running and Bruce Fordyce led the way, it wasn't considered unusual to take off along the roadside to stretch the legs. I didn't run religiously on leaving school or after my travels. Nor did I have any ambitions as a runner. It was just something I could do for myself whenever I felt like it.

When I started work in Johannesburg as a junior programmer, early in the eighties, I discovered there were three ways that people liked to spend their lunch breaks. Most stayed in the building and just headed for the canteen. Others took themselves to the pub, often in groups or even as a team-building exercise. I was invited to join my colleagues for a drink on a couple of occasions. I soon found it wasn't for me. In those days, pubs in the city tended to be located in basements. They were dark, cramped and dirty dives, not the kind of place where I felt able to relax.

Then there was a small number of people who used their lunch break as an opportunity to run. They'd bring their kit into work with them, change in the restrooms and then just take off. I'd see them heading out of the office or coming back. Each time I'd feel a pull. Eventually, I decided that was how I wanted to spend my free hour.

As running crept into my lunch hour routine, I began to look forward to the moment I could leave my workstation. It could be very hot and humid in Johannesburg for much of the year. Afterwards, I'd wash in the restroom basin. Still, I'd start the afternoon at work feeling reinvigorated and refreshed. In fact, I soon found that running was an excellent time to think through technical issues and come up with solutions. Once, I'd been snagged on a problem for days. I'd written the code and tested it, and even skipped lunch in a bid to find a solution. Every time, it tripped up at the same point and I could not work out why. I'd spend hours staring at the screen, go home and think about it over supper. I wasn't sleeping properly at night and would wake up each morning to find it uppermost in my mind. After another fruitless morning, I decided to finally take a break and vent my frustrations on a run. I went out fast and just submitted to the moment.

Then, as I pounded the walkways around the city's drive-in movie theatre and the spoil heaps from the gold mines, the solution sprang into my mind.

The moment I stopped thinking about it, and instead focused on the here and now, the answer that had been evading me materialized. Fearful that I might promptly forget it, I raced back to the office. Still dripping in sweat, I dropped into my seat and made one small change to a string of code. It worked perfectly. The relief was enormous, and I had one thing to thank for that.

When it came to running, I found that the rhythm and repetitive nature enabled a clarity of thought that I couldn't find so easily when stewing in front of my computer screen. From that moment on, my lunchtime outings also served as a problem-solving exercise. Whenever I snagged myself on code, I knew where to find the answer. Eventually, that hour became the high point of my day.

In banking technology, I had joined a profession that was undergoing a period of rapid evolution. Computer software and hardware upgrades were continually changing, and those who worked at that coal face were in high demand. I was young and ambitious, and it wasn't long before I found myself in a new post at another bank in Johannesburg with an increase in responsibilities. This time, the lunch-hour running culture attracted bigger numbers. From a workforce of 1,000, at least fifty went out regularly. Our offices also had a gym and proper changing rooms with shower facilities. With no more washing at the sink, it was one of the perks that led me to think I'd made the right move.

By now, my relationship with running was changing. It remained something I enjoyed and I found myself wanting to improve. I bought a basic digital watch that allowed me to time my runs. That soon became the focus of my hour. It gave me structure and incentive. I would also stretch the distance I ran from 5K to 8K. I liked the process of finding it hard and then progressively easier as my fitness improved.

In short, running had encouraged a competitive streak in me. I'd seen it in my brother at school, and now it seemed that it had found me, too. As a runner, however, I had only one rival. Every time I headed for the main entrance of the building in my trainers, I prepared to go into competition with myself.

I wanted to do well in my job. I also enjoyed coming back from my lunch run feeling as if I had put in my best effort. In my new workplace, I began to notice that many people tended to run in groups. It wasn't something I'd done before, but I was drawn to the idea. My work could be quite solitary and it seemed like a chance to socialize. In particular, I noticed one small group that always seemed so positive. The runners would smile and say hello whenever I passed them on the streets. They also ran with speed, grace and confidence, which made me think I could learn from them. I really wanted to be a part of that group. Firstly, however, I felt I had to get quicker for them to take me seriously. One time I found myself running behind them and it had been an effort to keep up. They had pace, which is what I set out to find before plucking up the courage to ask if I could join them.

After observing them for a while, I decided I would have to run a kilometre in under four minutes. At the time, this was quite a challenge for me. On my first few attempts, I finished woefully short and fighting for breath. Undeterred, I kept pushing at it every lunchtime. Within a week, I had broken that barrier. After making sure it wasn't a one-off fluke, and then finding myself in the changing room at the same time as the group as they prepared to go out, I braved enquiring if they could take on one more runner

'Of course!' said one, as if I didn't need permission.

In hindsight, I had set myself an unnecessary barrier. Running with that group, I quickly learned that what bound them wasn't speed but a sense of inclusivity. Anyone was welcome to join, and often the group would stretch out as some ran hard and others simply enjoyed the fresh air and the chat. In particular, I loved the fact that the group drew individuals from every department of the bank and from the lowest to the highest level. Status didn't matter. It was all about a shared love of the same activity. I made friends, but that didn't diminish my desire to improve. I admired those who were quicker than me. Inspired, I happily took up the invitation to join a team thrown together to represent the bank in a corporate challenge event. It was great fun, plus the race setting was a chance to compete against people who could push me. I saw it as an opportunity to start out as a beginner and then steadily learn from experience to become the best runner that I could be.

I was working in a job that I enjoyed, with prospects to grow my career. Just married, for the first time it felt like I was on solid ground. Life was good, and made all the more enjoyable by my deepening interest in running. It

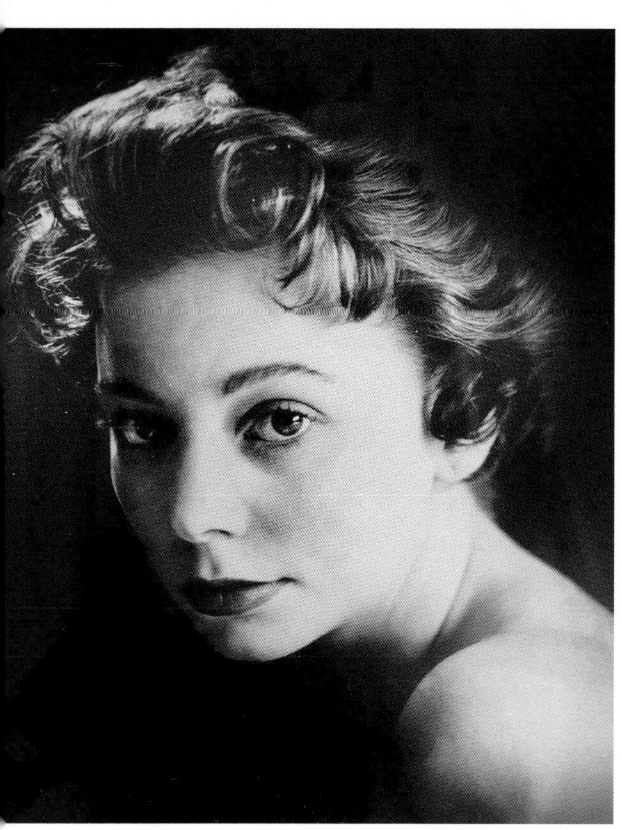

My mother, Mary Sinton-Hewitt, a woman who shone as a model in sixties South Africa but was largely absent from my life.

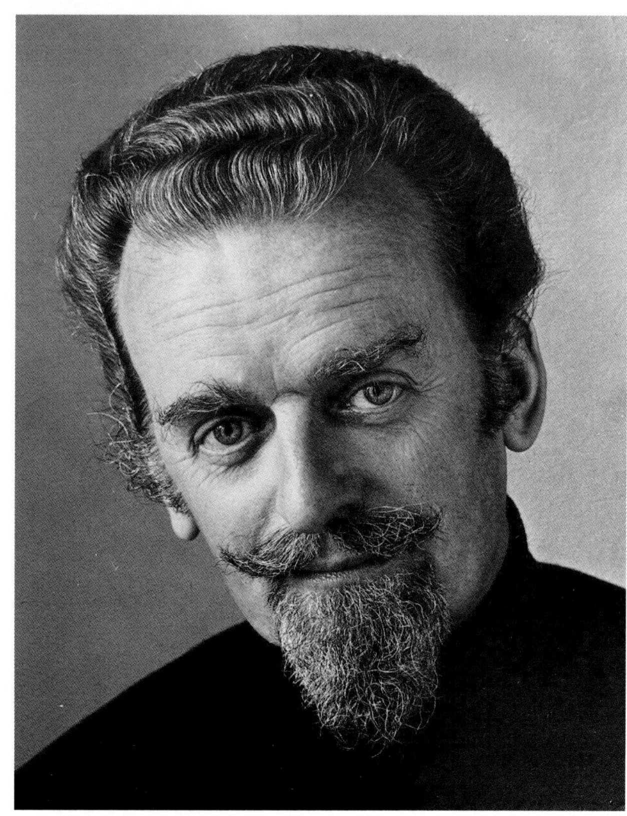

My father, James Sinton-Hewitt, a Scottish/Australian immigrant and photographer of note with a sharp eye for appearances.

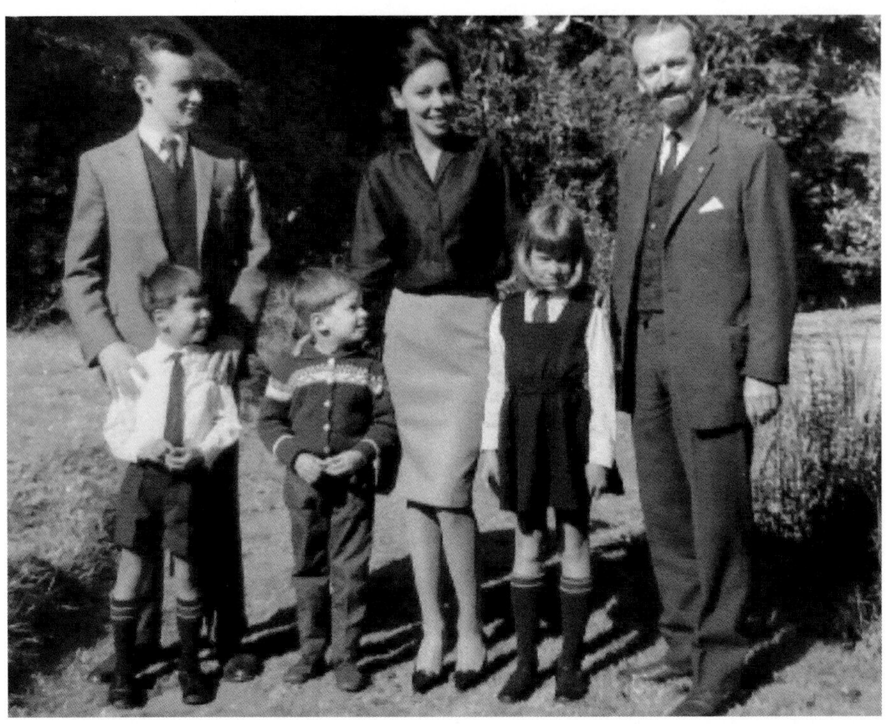

An early sixties portrait of the family before my mother left for the runways of Paris. Age four, I am standing between my sister Lindsay (right) and my brother Timmy (left), along with our older step brother, Noel.

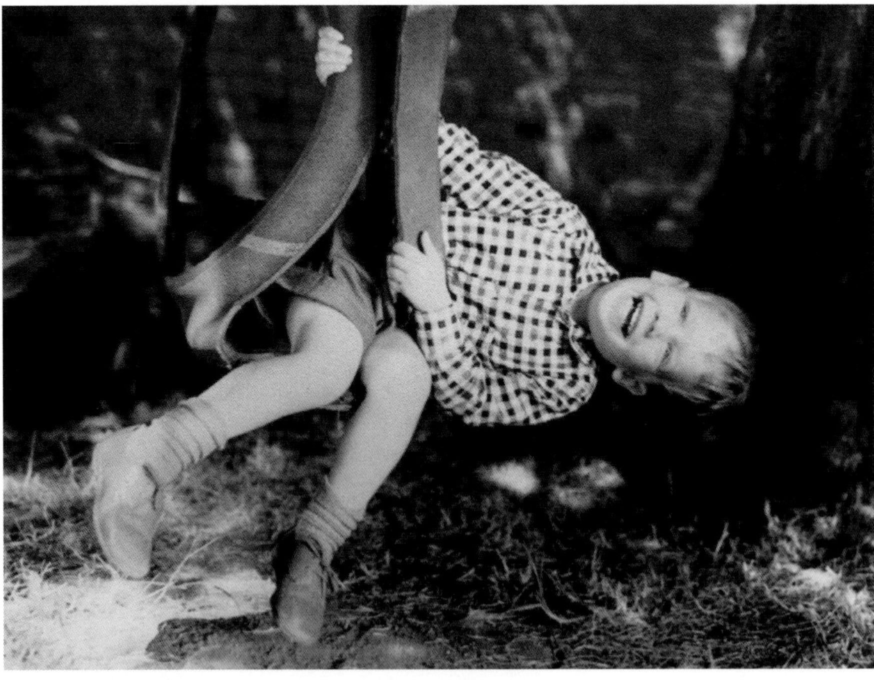

Playing in the garden beside the rondavel, a traditional hut common in South Africa.

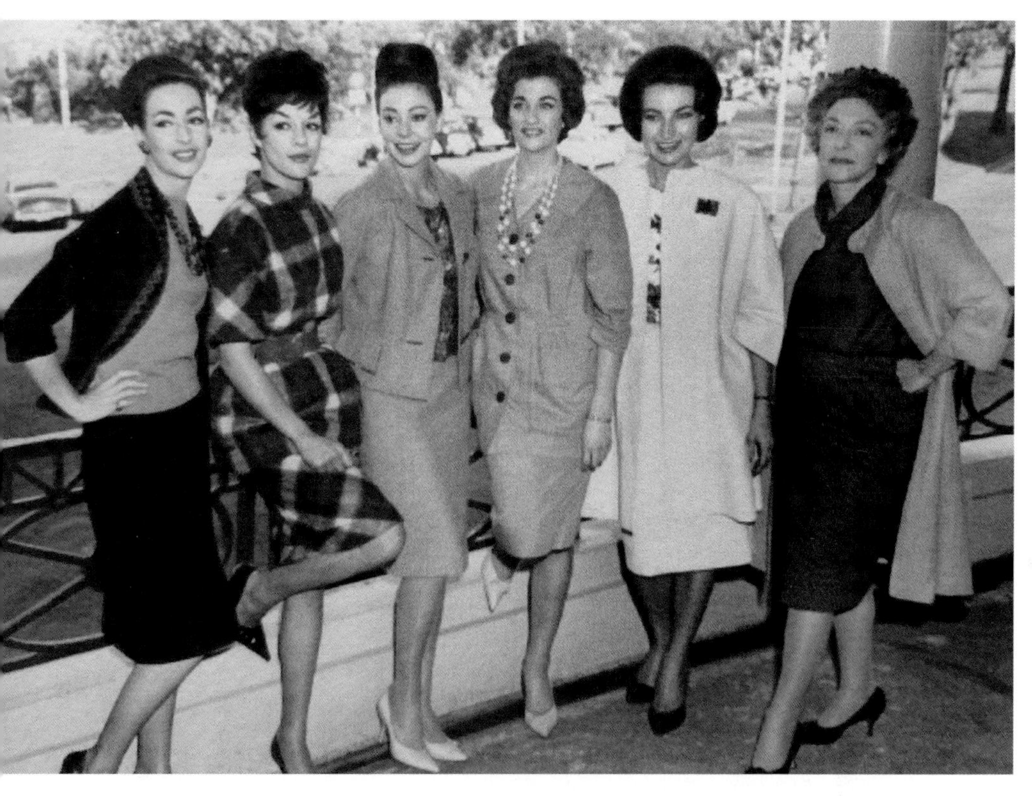

My mother (third from left), along with her modelling friends and their chaperone (far right).

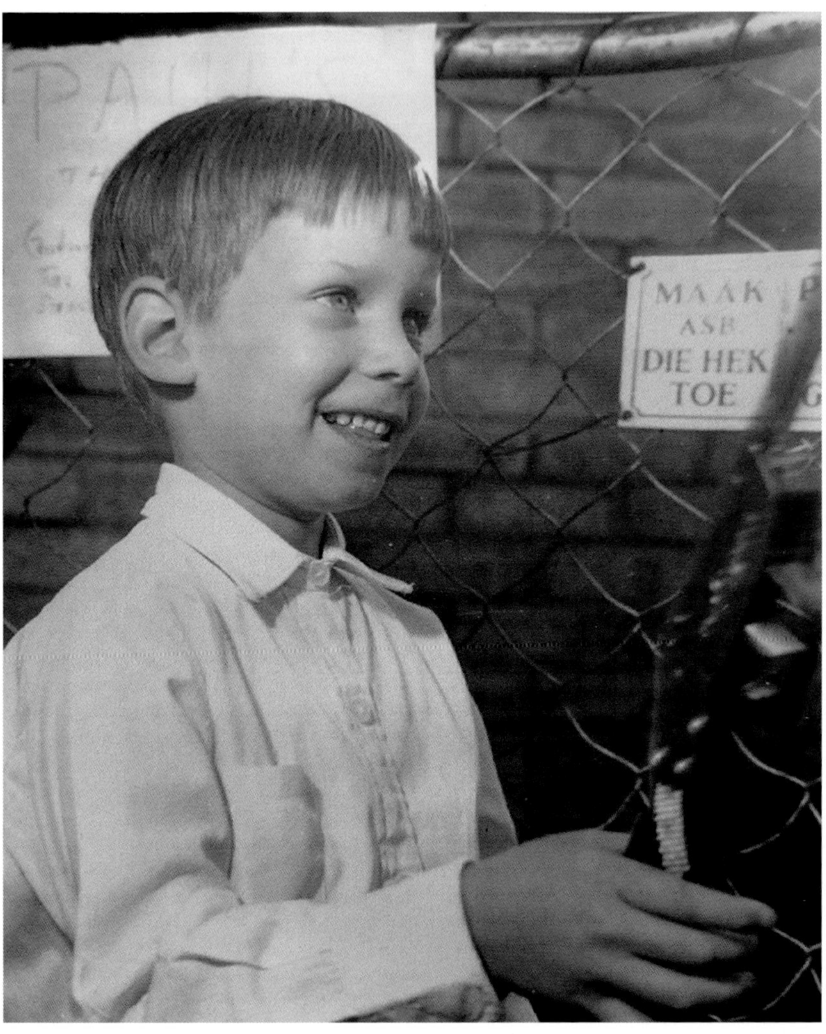

In the garden outside our house in Parktown North, Johannesburg, on my fifth birthday. Later that year, after our mother walked out on the family, my brother, sister and I would be placed into care.

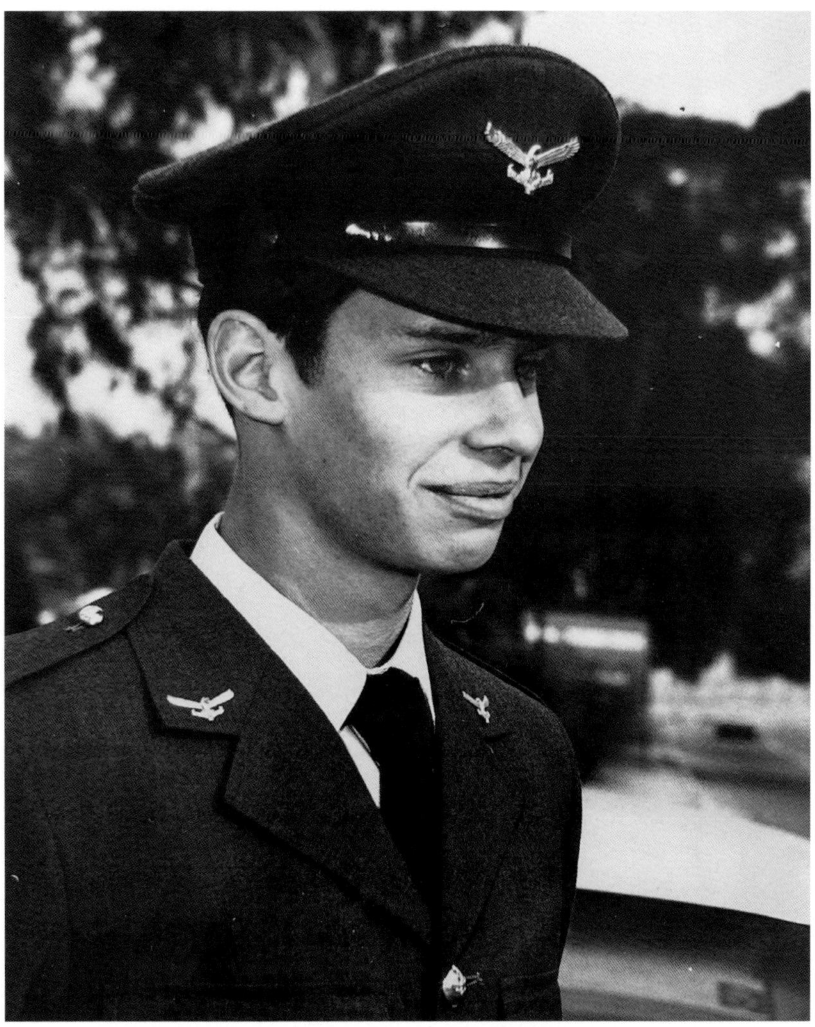

Lance Corporal Sinton-Hewitt reporting for duty!
At a time when conscription in South Africa was compulsory,
I served in the South African Air Force from 1979 to 1981.

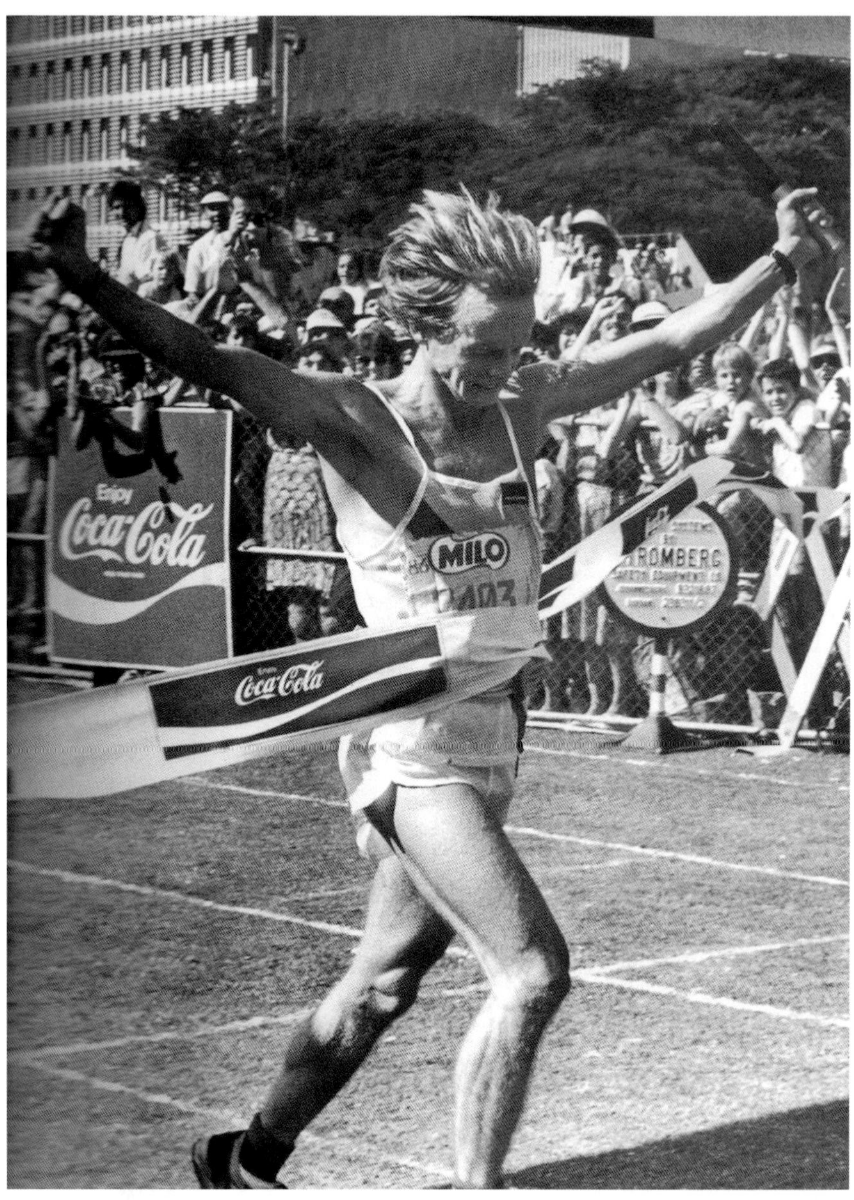

Bruce Fordyce crosses the finish line in one of his nine record-breaking Comrades Marathon victories, a streak that solidified his dominance from 1981 to 1990 as the greatest ultra-marathoner in the event's history. I served as a member of Fordyce's support crew on two occasions, which inspired me to chase my own running goals.

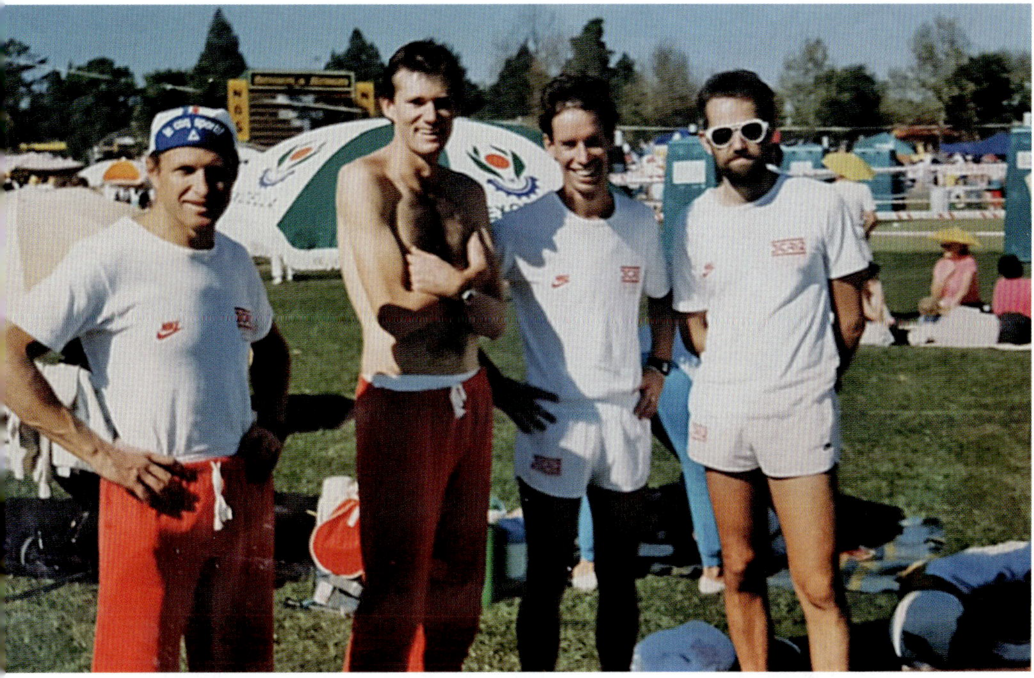

With my teammates at an interbank running event in the early eighties, including my colleague, friend and a pivotal player when it came to launching *parkrun* in New Zealand, Noel DeCharmoy (right).

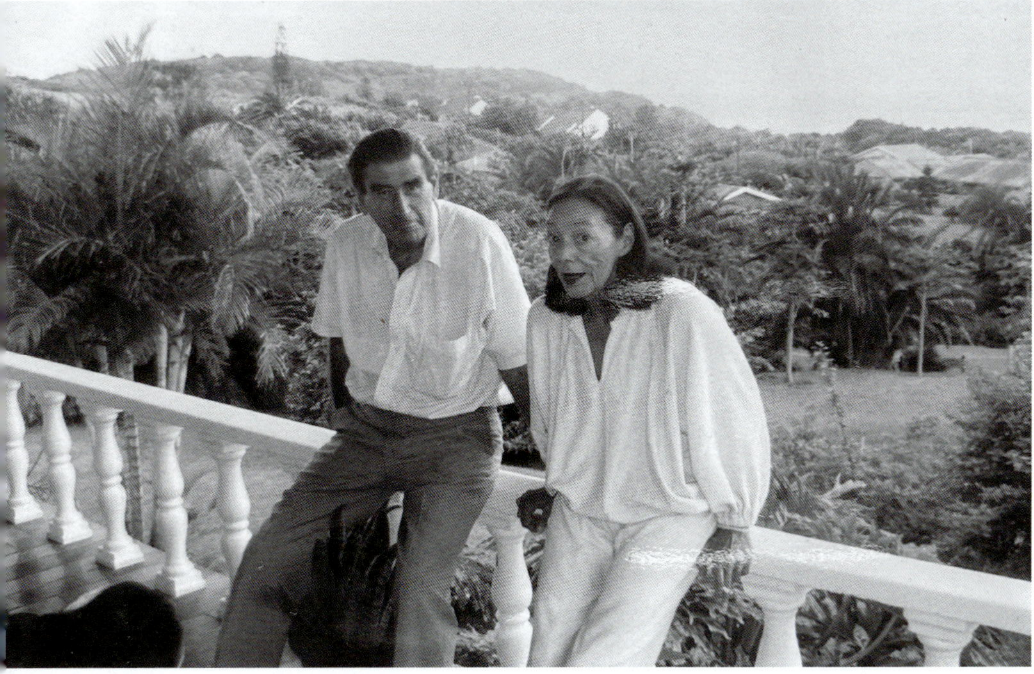

My mother with her second husband, Ian, in 1995 at their coastal home in Durban, South Africa. I took this photograph on a visit in which I hoped to find out why she had walked out on her family three decades earlier. It would be the last time I saw her.

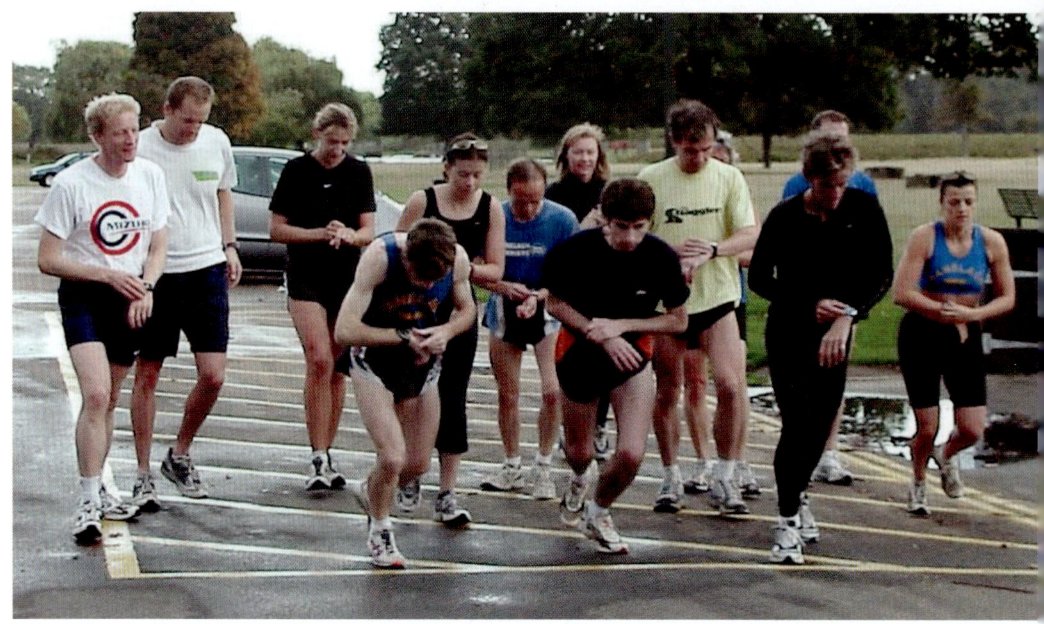

Thirteen '*parkrun* pioneers' on the start line for the first Bushy Park Time Trial in 2004. From left to right: Peter Wright, James Russell, Rachel Stanhope, Chris Owens, Karen Weir, Steve Rowlands, Tanya Wolken, Matthew Morgan, Andrew Lane, Julie Drummond, John Kipps, Simon Lawrence and Rachel Rowan.

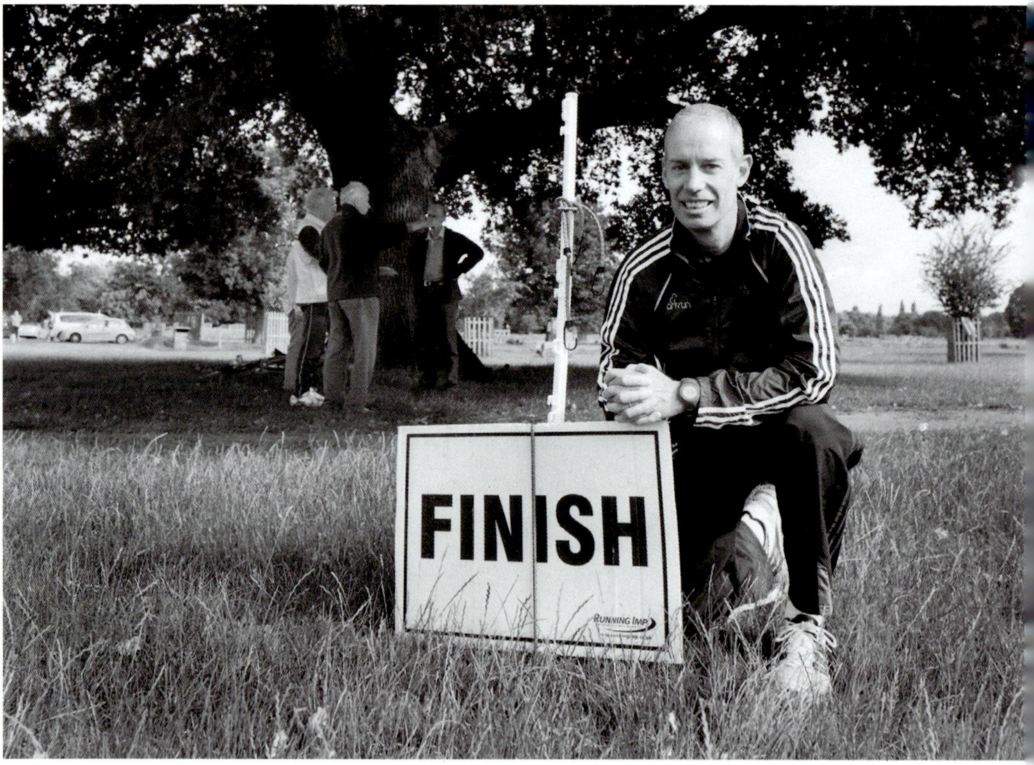

At the finish line seven years later to mark a partnership with Adidas.

became increasingly important to me. In work, I felt that I could relate to other members of my lunch-hour group more intuitively than others. Even if it was just a passing nod in the corridor, we had a common bond. Sometimes it felt as if running had become the lens through which I looked at the world, and that was fine by me. In my car, if I spotted someone out for a session on the pavement or the roadside I would note their form and estimate their pace.

Over time, running became a passion; an integral part of my identity. It meant so much to me, not least because I had chosen to bring it into my life after years of being told what I could and couldn't do. I tried not to dwell too much on my past. I kept telling myself that I had left it behind along with the institutions where I grew up. Only once did I feel drawn to revisit old times. It was a spur of the moment decision when I happened to pass through Parktown North one day. I had visited an external site for work, and the route back took me through the suburb where we first lived before the family fell apart. I couldn't drive on past the street that led to the little enclave at the far end we called home. As soon as I pulled off the main road, cruising between those neat, single-storey dwellings behind picket fencing, I felt transported. Everything seemed so peaceful, as if it existed in a bubble within a wilder world. As a little boy living there, I'd had no idea what lay ahead for me. I parked up and climbed out of the car, taking a moment to gather my bearings as if back from a long journey.

Our old house remained mostly obscured behind trees. The oak looked as magnificent as ever, while the jacarandas had climbed and spread in reach. Time hadn't stopped here as it had in my mind. The gate was closed, but I had no desire to venture further. I didn't want to know how I'd feel on the other side. I had come close enough.

As I turned to walk back to the car, happy I had taken this moment, a figure outside the house next door caught my attention. She was tending to a plant on her porch, unaware of my presence until I approached the foot gate.

'Mrs Freemantle?' It had been almost twenty years since I last saw our neighbour. She looked smaller, wiser, and just as kind. Looking across at me, she cupped her eyes against the sun and then rose to her feet. 'It's Paul. From next door.'

Recognizing my voice, perhaps, Mrs Freemantle beamed and threw her arms wide. As we greeted one another, I wondered how it must have been for those who knew my family when the children just disappeared. She grasped my wrists as she asked to look at me. I felt a little melancholy all of a sudden. It was lovely to see her. I just wished that someone had held onto me in the same way all those years ago.

'Come inside,' she said. 'I don't suppose Ann will recognize you!'

I vaguely remembered her daughter as a little girl before I was taken into care. It took me a moment to process that Ann had become the young woman who rose from the sofa to greet me. As for her boyfriend, with his wiry frame, long limbs and mop of blonde hair, I knew exactly who he was as soon as I set eyes on him. Even though he remained slouched on the sofa, I recognized that I was in the presence of running royalty. This was no figure from my past but from the here and now. In his values, achievements and ambitions, in fact, he represented so much of what I aspired to be.

'I'm Bruce,' he said as he reached up to shake my hand. 'Bruce Fordyce.'

14

ROCKY ROAD

My work in IT for the commercial bank mostly involved staring at screens. It didn't appear to bring any obvious transferable skills to support my efforts as a runner. Still, I found a way. It all came down to systems. Having grown up within one, I had emerged with a sensitivity towards processes. I saw life in terms of aims and outcomes. This helped no end in programming computers, which had evolved from punching holes in cards to represent a binary value to rudimentary software writing. It could also be very useful, I realized eventually, when it came to drawing up a training schedule to help me become a better athlete.

I just didn't know where to begin.

I had started out thinking I would just improve naturally. This proved to be true to an extent as I became fitter. Then I joined the group at lunchtime, and it became clear that a more structured approach to training would bring results. At school, the athletics team had pursued a set programme. I had just watched from the edge of the track with no real awareness of what that involved.

At home, I attempted to sketch out a timetable that I hoped would help me to improve. It was really just a spreadsheet that covered six weeks of running different distances. In terms of effort, I categorized each run as easy, tempo or hard, but without any sports science behind the formula. As I worked through my timetable, I saw vague indications that I was becoming faster. I just didn't really know why or how much further I could take things. Mostly I just enjoyed fiddling with data cells and numbers, as I did at work. I liked the analytical element, and hoped that eventually the goals I'd set myself would magically become reality. As I followed a process of my own making, so my time running went beyond a lunch hour session with my group to take in solo workouts. I was constantly pushing myself, inspired in the most part by runners in my cohort that I liked and admired.

In particular, I fell in with two guys who were both especially generous with their time and advice. Brian Chamberlain worked in the IT department, as I did. He was a quietly spoken man and highly observant. A details guy, he made small suggestions that could potentially make a big difference.

'Build in rest days for your body to recover,' he would say. 'Otherwise it's downhill all the way.'

There was another reason why I listened to Brian. As a runner, he had accomplished great things. If Comrades was the pinnacle of distance running in South Africa, the Two Oceans Marathon certainly rivalled the race in terms of prestige. Brian had won the race in 1977 and retained the crown in 1978, and on this basis alone it felt like a privilege that he was giving me his time and energy. Alongside him was the bank's chief accountant. Noel DeCharmoy had a sharp focus on numbers, and didn't hold back on his views about the schedule I had created for myself.

'Paul, this is bullshit,' he once told me, referring to some training block I had slung together on a spreadsheet, before suggesting how I could improve it.

Between Brian and Noel, the pair provided me with exactly what I needed. They understood how to assemble a training programme and tailor it to my personal needs. I also valued their advice and really appreciated the fact that they had adopted me as a work-in-progress. Above all, they gave me the confidence to feel as if the running community was one where I felt accepted.

As well as hitting the streets in their lunch hour, my two new friends were part of a running club associated with the city's university. Both were graduates which entitled them to lifelong membership. The pair were impressive athletes who took full advantage of the club's organized training sessions on a weekly basis. Keen to find any way to improve, I decided to take the step made by so many aspirational runners by joining a club of my own.

Rocky Road Runners is one of the oldest and most established running clubs in South Africa. Today, members still wear the distinct white vests with red, white and blue stripes across the chest. When I signed up, with some excitement, it certainly marked them out in the many inter-club races staged around Johannesburg. The 'Rockies', as they were informally known, had a rich heritage for producing distinguished runners. Their headquarters also happened to be close to where I lived, which was the deciding factor for me.

If my lunchtime group introduced me to a small band of people who shared my love of running, in the Rockies I found an entire community. The club catered for all abilities, but I found myself gravitating towards the faster groups because I wanted to learn from them. At the same time, I was becoming increasingly good friends with Noel and Brian. We'd meet up to run outside work, and I continued to soak in their wisdom and advice. My friendship with them also brought me into a social circle that soon involved the partners and families of the runners I had met. We would all gather for barbeques in the sunshine, and though we all came from different walks of life our friendships began from a shared love of the same activity. This was my tribe, I realized. No matter what the future held for me, I knew that running would always be at the heart of it. The performance aspect appealed to my awakening as a young man hungry to fulfil his potential, but above all it provided me with the sense of community that I had always craved. As runners we looked out for one another. So, when Noel invited me to join the race crew for a university club runner who had entered Comrades one year I jumped at the opportunity. For this wasn't any ordinary competitor but a legend of the sport.

I would be crewing for Bruce Fordyce.

The opportunity arose at the last minute. It was 1987. Bruce had won the race on the previous six occasions, with Noel on hand for several of those in a key supporting role. This included passing him food and tailor-made drinks as he ran to stay fuelled and hydrated, along with any information he needed about competitors' positions so that he could make tactical decisions. That year, to cover the 55-mile course, the crew consisted of six people on three motorbikes. I would be one of the pillion riders and the point of contact for Bruce at agreed points in the race.

My role was relatively simple but I couldn't afford to mess it up. A mistake could affect the outcome of Bruce's race, after all. A few days before the event, we gathered for a briefing at his mother's house in Johannesburg. Outwardly, Bruce was as relaxed as he had been when I met him by chance at the Freemantle house. He remembered we'd met, and though he was cheery and down to earth I remained in awe of him. As a runner, I felt like an apprentice in the presence of a master. Observing him at close quarters as the briefing unfolded, I noted how Bruce paid attention to every detail. He constantly asked questions about timings to be sure it would deliver. Collectively, we pored over the map to pinpoint where we would meet him and then hand over supplies on the move. Bruce was in good hands with a seasoned support crew member like Noel. I just wanted to show that Bruce could have every confidence in me too.

Come the day of the race, the Fordyce crew assembled long before dawn. I felt so nervous that I might as well have been at the start line with Bruce and all the other competitors. All I could do was stay warm until the sun came up on a bright, humid and testing day to run an ultramarathon. From the moment we set off on the bikes, just before the start of the race, I barely paused for breath.

Riding pillion behind Noel, I switched between map reading and navigation to reach our crew points in time. There, I would prepare to briefly run alongside Bruce to provide him with whatever he needed without costing him a second in pace.

'Who's behind me?' he asked, as I passed him a drink at our final handover. 'How close? What shape are they in?'

I was ready with the answers, having gathered the information as planned, which I delivered with the same precision as if I were responding to an officer back in the military. In that moment, it brought me close enough to recognize that Bruce was pushing through physical and mental exhaustion. His expression, tight with pain as much as concentration, spoke volumes about his focus and perseverance. Despite all the alarm bells sounding in his brain and body, in a race that would take him just over five and a half hours to complete, he maintained a metronomic pace. It was exciting and exhilarating, especially as it became clear that our runner was about to extend his reign as king of Comrades with another victory. As a measure of the popularity of the race, it was quicker for Bruce to reach the finish on foot than it was for us to negotiate traffic on the bike. We might not have made it in time to see him breast the tape, but we didn't miss out on the celebrations.

I was part of a winning team and a shared experience that meant so much to me. The victory brought competitor and crew together, as it did for us all the following year when Bruce won the event for the eighth year in a row, and who added a ninth on his final victory in 1990. In doing so, it felt like I could even consider one of South

Africa's greatest runners to be a friend. What struck me most about Bruce was the gratitude he showed for our efforts. A sponsored athlete, backed by Nike, he invited his crew to a celebratory meal a few weeks after the win where he gifted us all with the latest running shoe from the brand. For any runner at the time, these were considered a state-of-the-art prize when it came to performance. From there on out, inspired by the efforts I had witnessed that day, I wore my Pegasus trainers with pride.

A cut above everyday running shoes because of the groundbreaking, grippy tread pattern modelled on a waffle iron, and with the iconic Swoosh on the sides, my fancy footwear certainly drew attention when I ran in my lunch hour or with the club. I liked to think they helped me to run faster. In reality, I had a clearer understanding that if I was to fulfil my potential then I needed to continue putting in the work.

Everyone runs for different reasons, of course. As I began to get serious, time became my central focus. With my competitive streak in full flow, I entered local races at every opportunity. I developed a constant hunger to get quicker and recognized that could only come from solid training and determination. I also had two mentors in Brian and Noel. On their suggestion, I took advantage of a feature of the Johannesburg running club scene: the time trial.

'The stopwatch doesn't lie,' said Brian, when I asked what purpose it would serve.

Alongside the Rockies, several clubs hosted regular time trials that were open to everyone. These weren't races as such, but a chance for runners to assess performance over short distances. One club might stage a 10K every two to three weeks or so, while another put on a 5K or 8K. If I travelled around the city, it meant I could find one at least once every week or two and build it into my training schedule. Runners from the participating clubs could just show up at the start line, usually on quiet roads after work, and a club volunteer would be on hand to record our efforts. I'd always be in competition with myself, but it helped to have other runners around me. I grew to recognize faces and names while also learning what times they were capable of achieving. As well as enjoying the company, it provided me with another way to assess my performance. It was all very informal, but runners like me found the data invaluable. The clubs tended to publish the results in their monthly newsletters or in local newspapers, which I picked up eagerly. I would log my results, and use that to help project a target time for a race distance that was fast becoming the gold standard for me.

The marathon struck me as a magical challenge. You couldn't just run it and hope for the best, as you might when faced with a 5K or 10K. Stretching to 26.2 miles, it required a combination of physical training, mental preparation and also strategy for anyone to perform to the best of their abilities. Ultimately, it came down to a process. As the Rockies were preparing to select two runners to represent the club in a marathon taking place in Cape Town, I knew what I needed to do if I wanted to be considered. I had to work at becoming faster and also learn to feel confident at that distance.

I could also count on my friends to help me prepare to run my best race.

At Noel and Brian's suggestion, I approached the time

trial in one of three different ways. Firstly, I'd run one at a comfortable pace. The next time I'd set out to beat that time. Then, on the third run, I'd leave nothing left in my bid to get round as fast as possible. Pushing myself until it felt like my lungs would burst, it was a deeply unpleasant experience. I also recognized that this was a state that a runner had to endure and even embrace in order to improve. Every time I felt as if I'd gone too far, my mind and body seemed to adapt to the demands.

After rest and recovery, I found that my comfortable pace had quickened by a notch. Not just in the time trial but over longer distances. Having spent time around Bruce Fordyce, I knew he believed a key component of his endurance training involved running for hours at an effort he could easily sustain. Since Brian and Noel had also encouraged me to increase my weekly mileage, I would happily spend several hours trotting around Johannesburg at my newfound relaxed pace.

Over time, by combining the long, slow runs with the short, sharp punch of the time trial, my speed and endurance steadily improved. Every aspect of my training was undertaken with the Cape Town marathon in mind. There was competition for the club place, of course, and no guarantee I would make the grade. So, when it came to the qualifying race, a half marathon in Johannesburg, I called on all the work Brian and Noel had put into helping me to become a runner who could be proud of his achievements. From the start, I set out to inhabit that state of pain I had become accustomed to and then stay there until I crossed the finish line.

And it paid off.

I was thrilled when I found out I had been selected to represent Rocky Road Runners in Cape Town. Immediately, I shared the news with my two friends. It felt like a joint achievement, and one that we'd worked hard to earn. Together with one of the club's best runners, I flew to Cape Town in a state of excitement and much trepidation. I had prepared as well as possible, but was in no way winning material. My teammate left me for dust at the start line, and was soon jostling for position near the front, but that didn't matter to me. Even in a field of hundreds I was only ever racing myself, and that was fine.

For much of the race, I was alone with my thoughts. I fell into a rhythm and focused on checking off each mile-distance marker one after another. Mindful of the humid conditions, I made a point of grabbing a cup of water or coke from each aid table station. Even so, exhaustion crept into the last six miles and my pace began to slow.

'Oh, come on!' I muttered to myself, mindful of the effort I'd made to get this far. 'Not now!'

Even as the words left my mouth, my legs broke free from my resolve and I found myself walking. My head dropped in defeat. I felt like a failure. Maybe the marathon wasn't for me.

'Keep going.' I looked across to see a marshal in a tabard at the side of the road. She smiled and clapped her hands. 'You can do it.'

I smiled grimly, shaking my head as I passed her, but she didn't stop clapping and offering me encouragement.

Then, after no more than a couple of steps, I responded by picking up my pace. The marshal acknowledged it with a small cheer and I realized I was running once again. Not as briskly as before, but I was back in the moment and with a matter of miles to go.

I finished the race in 2 hours and 36 minutes. It was a little way behind my stellar teammate, but my result went beyond what I had hoped to achieve. I was delighted, and though I knew I'd wasted precious seconds in the final phase I had learned a great deal about myself as a runner. I'd always believed it was a solitary pursuit. Without those simple words of encouragement from the volunteer marshal, however, I might have dropped out completely. As well as earning me a medal and a personal best time, that race showed me how running could connect us in unexpected ways and bring out the best in everyone.

In many ways it was the experience that meant more to me than the result. It also helped to give me a sense of purpose. At a time in my life when I lacked the confidence and experience to do anything but conform to what I believed was expected of me, running showed me what was possible if I struck out on my own. By following a process, even if it was challenging, I could earn a shot at an outcome that might otherwise have been out of reach. Above all, in the last years of my life in South Africa before leaving for Europe in 1989, running was what made me happy. In those days, there was little understanding of the association between lacing up a pair of trainers and mental health. Until I faced a therapist many years later, the vocabulary just wasn't there. All I knew was that it could lift my mood, and sometimes it felt like the only way. Because away from running, having got married in the belief that it would lead to a more settled existence, my life was become increasingly more complex. I had a career and a young family, but both felt as if they were slipping from my control. Work was taking me onwards and upwards, and with that came professional demands and pressure to relocate. I was struggling as a husband and though I tried my best as a father it felt as though I had no template. Little things undermined my confidence, like the fact I didn't know any nursery rhymes because nobody had sung them to me as a child. I had a key role in a small family unit, something I'd craved my whole life, and yet my experience came from institutional living. Collectively, the guilt, doubts, stress and anxieties that my situation created felt like a weight on my shoulders.

Then I would go running, and it felt like a release.

15

FOOTPRINTS

Sometimes it seemed to me that it wasn't just marathon runners that could hit the wall. In life, even when we've come so far, things could still fall apart without warning.

It was counselling that got me back on my feet after the collapse of my marriage in 1995. The process encouraged me to revisit the milestones and examine them in a new light. The last thing I had expected to discover was my mother at the heart of it all. At first, I had found it incredibly hard to talk about her. Her behaviour throughout my childhood made no sense, but over time I came to recognize that only she could provide those answers. What mattered were the consequences, and through each session I would work towards some understanding.

My mother's withdrawal had left me feeling worthless. At first, it had encouraged me to occupy the sidelines of life. If she had walked away then clearly I didn't have much to offer, I told myself, while any attention that I drew usually spelled trouble. Over time, drawn by a yearning to belong, I had found a place in spaces where my value could be measured by achieving goals. My career was effectively defined by targets, as was my approach to running. I was constantly chasing deadlines in the workplace and improved times in races, all of which just masked the fact that my self-esteem was at a low. And if I had such a poor opinion of myself, as my counsellor had helped me to recognize as we unpicked my difficulties with relationships, how could I accept that others saw anything in me?

When the sessions came to an end, I left feeling as if perhaps I had the tools to get my life back on track. Having settled in the UK several years earlier, where my ex-wife and children remained, it felt like home to me now. I certainly had no desire to go back to South Africa. A few years before the break-up, and shortly after my first job outside the country had taken us to Belgium for a stint, I had moved the family back to Johannesburg. At the time, the apartheid system was crumbling at last. It could only be welcomed, but the transition to democracy was marked by a rising wave of racial, political and ethnic violence. Having spent time in the relative calm and order of Europe, and watching events unfurl on television, it came as a shock to find ourselves in the thick of such volatility and unrest. The country felt so claustrophobic. Everything seemed so much smaller and more intense. Killings were commonplace, and it seemed as if everyone knew somebody who had been stabbed or shot. We drove everywhere with our car doors locked, and if we had to stop at traffic lights we did so in a state of alert.

Within a year, I took the offer of a job in London and we got out of South Africa to start another new life. While the post took me another rung up the ladder, the travel demands added to the strains within the family. Like the country we'd left behind, my marriage had reached tipping point. The separation and subsequent divorce left me at an all-time low, and shortly afterwards I had reached out for professional help.

Without doubt, counselling helped me to understand myself. It also empowered me to address questions I had about my past. As the sessions progressed, I realized that only one individual could provide many of those answers. All we ever did was talk about her, and how her absence from my life had affected me. In order to complete the picture, I needed to face my mum.

'Just leave it alone, Paul. It's in the past. What good will it do?'

When I told my brother that I planned to visit our mother in Natal, he immediately reminded me of the position he had maintained since leaving South Africa. Tim understood my reasons for reaching out. He just didn't see the sense in setting myself up for disappointment.

'I need to try,' I reasoned. 'It has to be worthwhile.'

With my marriage over, and holiday entitlement from work that I had to take, this seemed like the most appropriate opportunity. I took on board Tim's sense of caution. It's just by now I knew that if I didn't pursue it then I would never be truly at peace.

My mother was in her mid-sixties. When I contacted her to ask if I could visit, she was as distant as she'd always been. Over the phone, she expressed surprise but offered no reluctance or enthusiasm. I finished the call feeling like someone who had booked an appointment. Several weeks later, having made the journey by plane and then taxi, I found her on the porch to her simple but tidy single-storey house on a track scuffed with sand from the beach. It was late summer in Natal; a time of languid sunlight and the roil of distant storms.

'Paul,' she said simply as I climbed out of the cab. 'Look at you.'

I hadn't seen Mum in years, but she still possessed the same poise that bordered on detachment. We greeted each other with a tentative hug that was cordial but with plenty held back in reserve. She felt slight in my arms, and when her two dogs bowled out to see me I worried they might knock her over. Her husband, Ian, appeared behind them, calling them to heel. We shook hands cordially before he took a step back as if to provide space for mother and son.

I stayed for two weeks. At first, it felt as if I had moved in as a lodger. It took a few days for us all to feel at ease with one another, and for me to become familiar with their routine and fall in with it. I would go for walks on a wind-blown beach with my mother and the dogs. She adored them both, and I couldn't help feeling as if this was the first time I'd seen such a strength of affection from her. We talked, of course, but my mother was very good at keeping conversations at a surface level. A small voice in my head kept urging me to just speak from the heart.

Why did you leave us? What possessed you to give up on your children?

I just couldn't bring myself to put the questions into words. My mother provided no such opportunity, of course.

Every time I steeled myself to open up about the real reason for my visit, a catch formed in my throat. As the days ticked by, I might well have found the courage to ask even though I knew her answers would be difficult to hear. What stopped me was an admission from her that I stumbled on inadvertently, but which dominated the rest of my stay.

'I've noticed you don't smoke any more,' I observed, a few days after my arrival. I was also aware that she hadn't once poured herself a drink. Indeed, the house seemed completely free of alcohol. 'Is this a new you?'

'Doctor's orders,' my mother said simply, as we walked along the compact sand just inside the high-tide line. 'They wouldn't operate until I did so.'

I stopped in my tracks and waited for her to face me.

'What operation?'

'I have cancer,' she said, as though that should have been obvious to me.

Her statement left me lost for words. I only came to my senses when she turned to continue walking with her dogs.

'You should have said!' I quickened my step to draw alongside her. 'When did you know? What kind? What stage?'

I had so many questions, but the answers were on her terms. My mother told me only that she was due for a consultation soon that would determine when the procedure could take place. When I asked if she had found it a challenge to give up the habits of a lifetime, at her doctor's insistence, she made it sound as easy as switching off a light. When she moved the conversation on to other matters, all I could determine was that she was a woman who sought complete control over every aspect of the situation. She told me Lindsay knew she was unwell, but as my sister hadn't shared the news with her brothers I guessed Mum had only disclosed half the story. The course of the illness was out of her hands and I imagine that terrified someone like her.

In the remaining time we had together, I came to realize I wasn't the only one to see through my mother's stoic facade. Ian was a loyal husband. His world revolved around her, which must have suited her down to the ground. He wasn't the type to break rank and tell me something she had refused to share with her own son. Even so, his vigilant attention wasn't lost on me. He knew full well that her illness wasn't something she could continue to outwardly ignore, and I appreciated how much he cared about her.

'You should consider visiting,' I suggested to my brother when I called to update him. 'There's no rush, but I think it might be serious.'

As the last day of my stay drew nearer, I was still mindful that I had questions that needed answering. Given that I now lived in the UK, I knew it could be the last time I saw my mother. If I didn't ask her now, I told myself, I might never have another opportunity. Having spent so much time in her company, however, I found that what still stopped me from addressing it had changed. I was no longer frightened that I was voicing something unspeakable. That it might snap the last threads of the relationship between a mother and her son.

Now, I had come to realize that my mother simply wouldn't understand the question.

Throughout my stay, in conversations about everything except my reason for being here, it dawned on me that Mum felt no sense of responsibility for abandoning us. She hadn't done it with our best interests at heart, as perhaps my father had as he tailspun into a breakdown. Nor had she started a new life to punish him, or even reject us. My mother recognized that Lindsay, Tim and I were her children, but she didn't possess a maternal bone in her body. It was just missing from her makeup. There was no sense of guilt or remorse. She'd simply moved on with no concept of the consequences left behind.

In some ways, by coming out here I had found my answers. The following day, as I said my goodbyes to Ian and then my mother, I knew I would have to learn to be at peace with it all.

I left with mixed emotions, but on the journey home I found myself looking increasingly ahead. My work in the UK had brought a whole new raft of responsibilities, all of which required complete commitment from me. I couldn't afford to be distracted, and in some ways the workload was just what I needed. Then there were my plans to spend more free time running. Having found the language to connect it to my mental wellbeing, I knew it needed to be at the heart of the next chapter in my life. I would be there for my mother, of course, but I left South Africa feeling like she didn't need me.

On the day that I landed back in London, my mother attended her scheduled consultation. She underwent a series of tests, scans and X-rays before the doctor in charge of her treatment called her in to discuss the next steps. It soon became clear that the proposed operation was no longer viable. The cancer had spread so rapidly that the remainder of my mother's life could be measured in weeks if not days. In view of this bleak, shocking news, and the complications she faced, the doctor recommended that she would be most comfortable in a hospice. There, her palliative care could be properly administered and she would be free to prepare in whatever way felt appropriate to her.

'We can make this happen today,' said the doctor, who had been careful to soften the urgency behind the situation without masking the reality.

My mother, always the model, was adept at putting on a front. Despite the inevitable shock, she kept her composure and moved to retain some command over the time she had left.

'Next week,' she insisted. 'And not before.'

Back home, my mother had a conversation with her devoted husband, the details of which would be known only to them. Given the consequences, I can only think she called on her lifelong skill in shaping an outcome to put her needs before anyone else. At some point during that weekend, she and Ian gathered their two dogs and bundled them into the car in the garage. The couple duly climbed in after them and started the engine, but not before attaching a hosepipe to the exhaust and feeding it into the vehicle's interior.

If Mary had to go, it would be on her terms.

It was my sister who called me with the news. A friend had visited my mother's house. When nobody answered, she investigated the sound of an engine running behind the garage door. My mother and one of the dogs were dead. Ian was unconscious and rushed to hospital, and the surviving dog taken on by the neighbours. I flew back to South Africa with Tim, feeling wretched that I had told him there was no urgency to visit. Of course, what happened was something nobody could have foreseen, but the guilt just added weight to my numbness and grief.

Physically and emotionally, poor Ian never fully recovered. Some years later, alone with a pistol, he fulfilled what his late wife had asked of him. It brought no closure. Just a sorry end to a relationship with a woman who had grown up barefoot and then trailed footprints through life that would leave the people who loved her feeling lost.

16

DOG DAYS

Throughout the years that followed, running became the thread that held my life together. In work, as a father and as someone still seeking to find a way to fit in, it could sometimes feel as if things were coming apart at the seams. My career in computer technology evolved into a marketing directorship in the same sector. It took me from the back rooms of commercial banking to system design for data networks. I spent much of the late nineties shuttling between the UK and the US, flying high, but ultimately it was redundancy that brought me back down to earth.

At a time when technology was in a state of rapid evolution, I took up a senior leadership role with a tech startup. We had just arrived in the first decade of the new millennium. In 2001 and 2002, innovators could become millionaires if they positioned themselves in the right time and place. The sector also attracted venture capitalists seeking crazy returns, and when that failed to happen they took flight overnight. Once again, I found myself without work.

With a mortgage to pay, and in a period when my two teenage children along with their dog would stay at the house as a London base, I had to find work fast. The industry I worked in was becoming increasingly crowded, however. Having only recently turned forty, I was beginning to think I might be too old for the marketplace. With my confidence diminishing, and my anxiety rising, I took the first job in the sector that I could find. After going from writing code to marketing the product, I now found myself in the business of selling it. I had no prior experience in this role, which involved driving up and down the country to meet potential buyers. I swiftly realized I didn't love it. Success in this field required a confident, brash and ballsy personality, and that really wasn't me. I worked hard at it. I just couldn't see myself in it for the long haul.

The same could be said of my experience with dating and relationships. Since the divorce, feeling as if I might be eternally lonely, I had made every effort to meet someone new. I'd been on dates that had developed into romances, and yet on every single occasion they ended the same way. Just as things were shaping up, I would look ahead and back out. I had an awareness of what was causing my commitment issues thanks to the counselling I'd received. As a result of my upbringing, and the heartache of a marriage that had hit the rocks, I couldn't hold onto the belief that I had what it took to make things work. It left me torn. I craved companionship, only to panic when I found it and cause more misery all round.

Caught in a cycle of constantly getting burned, it took a while for me to realize that I was the one who was starting the fires.

Amid this turmoil and uncertainty, I had just one means of finding calm and certainty. As a runner, work and parenting commitments largely dictated just how much time I could spend pounding the pavements and the parks in my neighbourhood. I tended to carve out space at the end of the day to decompress after hours stuck behind the wheel of a car. In South Africa, I had been driven by a competitive urge. I hadn't lost that, but while I tried to navigate life it dropped down my list of priorities.

Above all, I enjoyed the fact that running connected me with people outside my life at work and home. Thinking back to the opportunities I had found with the Rockies in Johannesburg, I joined a local club near my home in Twickenham. With an emphasis on the social side of running, the Stragglers brought me into the orbit of men and women who became good friends. At the weekly club run, where we met at the local YMCA and then split into groups, I fell in with a guy at a stage in life similar to mine. Duncan Gaskell was recently divorced and rebuilding his life having moved down from Yorkshire. He worked in sports management, which I found fascinating. Duncan was also a very good runner. He was a little older than me, and a little quicker. Deep down, that needled me in the best way possible. It reminded me that while times weren't my priority in that moment, the drive to push myself was still there. Like me, Duncan enjoyed the social opportunities that the Stragglers created. Together in those group sessions, we would jog side by side and set the world to rights. Before long, we were joined by another runner who I came to consider a close friend. Jim Desmond worked with computer systems, which reminded me how much I missed that field before marketing and then sales crept into my career. He was driven by data and details. So, when we talked about running in terms of pace and performance, Jim could reel off figures to add depth to the discussions. I loved our conversations during those sessions, and they would invariably broaden over a beer with other club members at the YMCA bar.

The regular runs and club events even served as an informal dating network. It was only a matter of time, of course, before my track record for detonating relationships without good reason caught up with me. Having broken up badly with a Stragglers runner I had been seeing for some time, causing a conflict of loyalties among our mutual friends, I felt obliged to leave the club. It didn't take me long in my guise as a travelling salesman to feel like I'd lost something important to me. With long, solitary days in the car, questioning how my career had brought me here, I realized how much I missed the camaraderie of my running friends.

As a Stragglers runner, I would often represent the club in local races, such as 10Ks and half marathons. I still liked to make an effort, even though my training wasn't geared specifically towards performance. We often competed against a neighbouring club called Ranelagh Harriers. They took things far more seriously, and would often produce runners who finished on the podium. Finding myself in the mix with the Ranelagh runners in their blue vests, I would purposely put the hammer down just to dispel the myth that our club was all about chatting at the back of the pack. There was always something rewarding about seeing the surprise on their faces when a Straggler took them down on the line. It wasn't big or clever, but could be really satisfying. It also reminded me that I could still run a decent time if I worked for it.

Towards the end of my time with the Stragglers, I took part in the Kingston Marathon and set out to see what I could do. With a healthy respect for the distance, I had found time to put in some basic training. I was fit but only in a rudimentary way. On the day, it was great to have Duncan Gaskell supporting me by riding alongside at key moments to hand me drinks and offer encouragement. With no pressure on me, it was one of those races in which I felt good from the start. I was careful not to overcook things, and then spent the latter stages picking off competitors as they faded, including several blue-vested runners. It wasn't all plain sailing. Fatigue caught up with me in the last three miles. Duncan picked up on my drop in pace and urged me to push. In between swearing at him and feeling like I might faint, I reminded myself that I had hit the wall around this stage once before and it had almost cost me my race. My time wasn't all that important to me. I just wanted to say to myself that I had been in charge of my pace the whole way. With this in mind, I pushed hard for the finish line. That closing phase was a mental battle as much as a physical fight. It was often where the real test of the marathon began. Afterwards, when I finally picked myself off the ground, it was such a thrill to learn I had finished in third place. I was just five minutes off my personal best, with a time of 2 hours and 41 minutes.

Given that I hadn't set out to do anything more than enjoy myself, it felt like a solid achievement.

At the same time, in the recovery period that followed, a little voice in my head began to question how I might have fared with proper preparation.

From that moment on, my competitive spirit rose back to the surface. And so, on leaving the highly social Stragglers, with reluctance but knowing it was the right thing to do, it wasn't long before I went next door to the club that ran to race.

The group session with Ranelagh Harriers still provided me with an opportunity to meet people and make friends, but the pace quickened until nobody talked. It was hard work. It was also rewarding. After a year on the road as a salesperson, I was absolutely ready to focus on my performance as a runner. At the very least, the training process would serve as a healthy distraction from work. With the renewed attention I was paying to form and pace, it wasn't long before I began to question whether I could challenge a marathon time I had set at the outset of my running career.

Some fifteen years had passed since I ran a personal best in Cape Town. In that time, work and family commitments prevented me from seeing if I could better it. I was older, which counted against me, but now I had experience on my side. Having only been a little slower at Kingston, I figured I had set myself a baseline time to improve upon. If I could shave off just another six minutes, it would take me inside the magic mark of two and a half hours. Even though it didn't sound like much over 26.2 miles, I knew enough to recognize that it would take me to the limit of my physical ability. To stand any chance of success, I would have to put in a great deal of work. It meant no longer running purely for fun but committing to a training regime that would help me to sustain a demanding pace required on the day. With work sapping my soul, I was ready to invest the time and energy into maximizing my chances of success.

Above all, I wasn't getting any younger. Unless I committed to it now then I risked leaving it too late.

'Tim, are you ready to run? Let's go . . .'

I met plenty of potential training partners at my new club. I just found that my free time during the week was dictated by whatever time I arrived home from work. It was haphazard, which meant I couldn't make arrangements with anyone outside of the club sessions.

Instead, I found a running companion in the form of a dog.

The springer spaniel that my son brought with him to live with us, and who remained with me after he moved on to university, happened to share the same name as my brother. It was one of those coincidences that seemed both amusing and odd to me at first, and then perfectly normal. My brother, Tim, was not a runner. His namesake perked up just as soon as I appeared at the foot of the stairs in my shorts, shirt and trainers. Together, we would head for Bushy Park, a huge expanse of open heath, woodland and waterways, and which was also home to herds of roaming deer. While I did most of the talking with Tim the dog at my side, I was quite content in his company. He was such a good boy when it came to sticking beside me. If we detoured along the path beside the River Thames I could trust him not to divebomb the ducks.

It was a special time. I was doing something for myself, with a dog who just loved to be outdoors. If life felt like a treadmill, this was my moment to jump off and set my own pace and direction. When it came to the training plan, which for me took the form of a spreadsheet, I found I could put together the components with some confidence. I knew what worked for me, and the markers that I needed to hit as I worked towards a race the following year that I had always wanted to run. The 2004 London Marathon would be the twenty-fourth edition of the event. It was rapidly establishing itself as a major fixture in the world's sporting calendar. If I was going to achieve my goal of running a sub two-thirty time, I felt it would be fitting to do so here at a prestige event in my adopted home.

I had set up my running schedule to progress from a base level of fitness from autumn and through winter, before it ramped up considerably into the new year ahead of the race in April. By then, I intended to be in peak condition, not just physically but also mentally. Work wasn't ideal, and I certainly relied on my friends to stave off loneliness, but the wisdom of age and some stability in my life had at least brought a degree of calm. I wasn't running away from anything this time. I was aiming for a goal. Aware that this could be my last real shot at a new personal best marathon time, I certainly wasn't lacking in commitment and determination.

Whenever I had the chance, I always took part in club training with Ranelagh. It was a good way for me to find myself among runners who could push me. I also still ran with some of my friends from the Stragglers, notably Duncan and Jim. Between them, their companionship reminded me of my younger days when Noel and Brian first helped to bring me up to speed. At weekends, we would often all take part in local races. The rivalry was fierce but always good-natured. I loved that running brought people together from all walks of life. It struck me as a great leveller with little to stop anyone from joining in. All you needed was a pair of trainers and a dash of motivation, and it opened up a whole new world.

In my time with the Stragglers and then the Ranelagh Harriers, I made so many new friends who shared the same passion as me for running. It was the one thing we all had in common, no matter what our background or ability, aims and ambitions, and encouraged bonds to develop and deepen. It helped me get out of the house, built my social confidence and helped me to stay healthy in every way.

Then, just as my grand training plan ramped up for the London Marathon, and with only one goal in mind, I met a runner who would stop me in my tracks.

17

DANCE LIKE NOBODY'S WATCHING

As a runner, I was comfortable with myself. I could be quick by comparison to others in the club. I had even used my collective results over the years to calculate that I could place myself roughly within the top 5 per cent of most races. At the same time, I recognized that it was all relative. Whether other people were faster or slower than me, all that mattered was how I measured up against my own expectations. Counselling had opened my eyes to the fact that I tended to measure my value by setting goals. I was quite comfortable with that because frankly it served as an effective motivator. When I ran with a finishing time in mind, I just wanted to know that I had done everything correctly in my preparation and execution. By following the process set out in my training plan, I could be calm, positive and confident in my outlook.

It was a far cry from how I felt in my role as a software salesman. Chasing leads and attempting to close deals, I rarely felt anything but stressed and anxious. I loved the sociable side of my life. It's just for all the friendships I'd made through running clubs, something I valued because it felt like I'd missed out on those connections while growing up, my dating history chipped away at my self-esteem. Given my instinct to back away from commitment, believing I was damaged goods, I became reluctant to venture into that territory at all. It wasn't ideal and I felt lonely at times. I just didn't want to risk hurting anybody.

It was all the more reason for me to focus my energies on training. I was committed to the process, and the steady improvements in my performance helped me to feel fulfilled. Even so, in running up to 80 kilometres a week – and sometimes pushing it to 100 kilometres – I was spending a lot of time alone with my thoughts. I would reflect on my lot in life, and began to wonder what I could do to improve those areas where I felt unfulfilled. While I resigned myself to the fact that it would take a miracle for me to find someone special who would want to share my life, I came to realize I had the power to steer my career back on course.

Barrelling up the motorway one day, on my way to another pointless pitch, I reached the conclusion that my time as a system software salesman was coming to the end of the road. I had no passion for it, which was starting to drag me down. Having been so determined to climb out of a dark place following the collapse of my marriage, I knew that something had to change to stop me from sinking again. I reminded myself that I had twenty years of experience in development and also marketing. That had to be worth something.

Towards the end of 2003, I began to quietly make enquiries among my contacts in the tech sector. My efforts resulted in an opportunity to join a small software team developing a search tool. The role on offer excited me, which was something I hadn't felt at work for a while. It was enough to persuade me to hand in my notice as a salesman and prepare to restart in the new year. It also meant I had a short period in which I could prioritize my marathon training. In that time, thanks to the progress I was making with my running programme, I was brimming with self-belief. I carried that positivity through the Christmas break and then used it to start my new job determined to make an impression.

Within a matter of weeks, I could safely say that I had achieved just that.

Keen to position myself as a key player, just as my new employer expected from me, I had taken it upon myself to write and distribute an internal evaluation paper about the potential of the algorithm behind the company's search engine product. In doing so, I set out to explain how it functioned so that anyone within the organization could understand. I also pulled no punches about its potential in this highly competitive new tech sector, believing a frank assessment would lead to improvements and ultimately growth. Instead, my new boss was so enraged at what he considered to be a hit job from within that he fired me on the spot.

It all happened so quickly that it left me in a state of shock. I had presented the paper with the best of intentions, unaware that such honesty was the last thing the company's chief executive wanted to hear as he sought to attract investors. Despite my self-confidence deserting me as I received my marching orders, my immediate response was to find another job as quickly as possible. Even without this disastrous, short-lived spell on my CV, however, I found myself waiting in vain for the phone to ring. Nobody, it seemed, was interested.

The same thing could be said for my love life.

Essentially, I was looking for someone who could help me to overcome all the obstacles to a relationship that I had created for myself. It was beginning to feel like that person didn't exist. Among my friends at Ranelagh Harriers, it was no secret that I was single, but perhaps in need of some informed matchmaking. Had such help been offered to me directly, I would have been mortified and refused on the spot. Knowing this, a friend at the club quietly put together a plan without me or the individual in question having any idea that we were about to be set up.

I had met Jo once before. Another Harrier, she had been one of a group that had gone to lunch after a weekend race the previous year. I was late in joining them, and found myself taking the only chair available, which was opposite from where she was sitting. Jo was a tall red head with a kind smile and quick sense of humour. A psychiatric nurse, she was recently divorced and a parent of two children. It gave us something in common, but we quickly found it easy to talk to one another about every subject under the sun. I liked Jo a lot. It's just having crawled to the running club from the wreckage of a relationship at the Stragglers, I had no intention of being anything but polite, friendly and reserved.

I can only think our mutual friend had noted us chatting and seen something there that she couldn't ignore. Like me, Julia had a place at the London Marathon. She was running for charity, and in order to raise funds had arranged to host a salsa night for club members. I didn't consider myself to be an enthusiastic dancer, and having just lost my job I hardly felt like I could be the life and soul of a party. Still, I was happy to make a fool of myself once in a blue moon if it was for a good cause.

'Jo is here,' said Julia, having made a beeline for me when I arrived at the hall she'd hired for the event. 'She's on her own, so make sure you look after her.'

I didn't read anything into the request. I was also completely unaware that earlier Julia had briefed Jo that I would be alone and grateful for the company. So, when we found each other on the sidelines, both Jo and I assumed we were just helping out the party host.

'Do you dance?' she asked as the evening got underway, and promptly grabbed my wrist in such a way to make me think there could be only one answer.

While my default would be to hold back, I was happy to let go in the right company. I certainly felt relaxed with Jo, and together we laughed a lot as the salsa teacher put us all through our paces.

That evening, we danced together until the hall lights came on. Any sense of reserve that I might have hidden behind fell away. My salsa technique left a great deal to be desired, but I felt so relaxed in Jo's company that I didn't care what anyone else made of this lanky guy flailing his limbs about on the dance floor. It was a joyful time marked by much laughter. Jo mesmerized me. Straight away, I knew that I had met someone special.

It was the last thing I expected in my life at that moment. Having just found myself without work, however, it left me unsettled. As I signed up to agencies and waited for a break, I began to question what I could offer this relationship. Sure enough, it stirred up all the familiar anxieties. Jo was incredible. She represented everything I could wish for in a partner. She was kind and loving, funny and outgoing and an amazing mother to two children. Jo was nothing but understanding about my work situation. I still felt raw about what had happened, but she encouraged me to stay positive. Then there was my marathon preparations, which had become as important to me as flotsam to a shipwrecked sailor. To anyone else my training regime must have appeared deeply uncompromising. Jo just took it in her stride. An accomplished runner in her own right, and sensitive to my situation, she seemed to instinctively understand what it meant to me. I was committed to the training plan, and yet when it came to the relationship I kept doubting my place in it.

My misgivings had nothing to do with Jo and everything to do with me. I had grown to care for her very quickly, and we were spending a lot of time together. Inevitably, I began to look ahead at the possibility of some kind of life together and the panic would set in. The last thing I wanted to do was lead her down that path in case I could offer her nothing at the end of it. Jo had children, after all, and I knew how much they needed stability. Even though Jo helped me to feel complete, I couldn't shake off the belief that I could never be enough. With this in mind, and having somehow convinced myself that I was doing the decent thing, I dropped round to break the news to Jo.

'So, I think we should call it a day,' I said, finding no good time to raise the moment over a cup of tea. 'But I'm hoping we can still be friends.'

Cup in hand, Jo regarded me over the rim.

'I don't need any more friends,' she said firmly, and in a way that made me think that although she was quite calm an anger had just ignited inside her. That she showed no sign of shock also suggested that my reputation for breaking off healthy relationships had followed me from the Stragglers. 'You'd better leave then.'

Almost immediately after Jo closed the door behind me, I regretted my decision. I was just following the same self-destructive process that had scuppered all my relationships. It had come up in counselling, and yet now I had just walked away from someone who genuinely made me happy. In hoping to minimize upset by getting straight to the point, I had also ended up being abrupt in a way that suggested I didn't care. Skulking home, I justified it to myself as proof that if I hadn't disappointed her then it would only be a matter of time. Jo deserved better than someone like me, as I had just demonstrated. My fear that I wasn't worthy of commitment had come to rule my life. It left me thinking that perhaps I was always meant to be alone. As someone who valued the company of others after such a lonely upbringing, I only had myself to blame for feeling quite bleak in that moment. Inevitably, word spread among the Harriers that Jo and I had split up. Almost everyone who spoke to me about it struggled to understand my reasons. The general consensus was that I had made a mistake.

And I agreed with them.

Jo and I still got along, even if it was uncomfortable in the aftermath, but gradually that unease made way for more practical discussions about the situation. The fact was that we still liked each other enormously. I recognized that I had detonated something that was potentially good for us both. I just couldn't see how we were able to move forward. As Jo saw things, however, my self-doubts were something only I could overcome.

'There is a way,' she suggested. 'If you genuinely want us to be together then embrace the thing that most frightens you. Take a step, Paul, and keep talking to me.'

Immediately, I knew that we both had the same thing in mind. We lived close to each other, and had divided our time between our two houses. Moving in together was a big ask, but having come close to self-sabotaging the relationship I wanted to prove that it had shown me what I stood to lose. Being out of work remained a huge source of concern for me. It brought financial worries and an anxiety that I'd scuppered my career. Despite knowing how fragile my mental health could be at times, I found that Jo's calm presence helped me to believe that I could get on top of that situation. We decided that my place was the better option for us to start this new life. With four children between us, in a two-up, two-down terraced house, it could be a squeeze at times, but soon proved to be a happy place. While my son and daughter were on the cusp of independence, and still staying with me on occasion, they were brilliant with Jo's kids and helped them both to settle in. It had been some time since I'd lived with the chaos that young children bring, compounded by a dog in the mix, but I surprised myself at how much I enjoyed it. Above all, I was so grateful to Jo for allowing me to prove to her and to myself that we could be stronger together. As that special someone I doubted could exist, she would transform my life. In encouraging me to discover that commitment was nothing to fear, but could in fact be an enriching experience if I shared how I was feeling, she had been forgiving of me, bold and generous.

Now it was on me to show Jo that I could go the distance.

18

STUMBLE AND FALL

In that early phase of 2004, running had seen me through several twists and turns. I'd lost my job and started looking for another, fallen in love and then filled my house with bedlam, laughter and joy. It seemed to me to be something that would remain with me forever. Having been my lifeline for twenty years, running provided me with space to think and find perspective, while also furnishing me with goals like the one that was looming on my horizon.

As the London Marathon approached, I felt as if I was close to being in the best shape of my life. I was in my early forties, but matching the pace I had achieved as a young runner. I just had to stick with the programme, follow that process, and give myself every chance of edging within the magical two-and-half-hour mark. In terms of my training, I was approaching the finish line. My challenge was finding the time for it as life became increasingly hectic. While running was an escape of sorts, the search for work had become my priority. I was living off savings but ultimately that was borrowed time. I'd spend my days applying for vacancies, making enquiries or meeting head-hunters. Then I'd switch into parent mode alongside Jo before seizing what remained of the evening. Whether I was running with Tim the dog, with friends or the club, I always made sure my time on feet was structured according to my marathon schedule. From a threshold or tempo session to hill repeats or a recovery run, I trusted in the process that would deliver me to the marathon start line knowing that I had ticked every box.

My training plan had started in the summer. In my mind, however, it extended back to the moment I completed the marathon in Cape Town some two decades earlier. I had never really appreciated my finishing time because I'd hit the wall. That had annoyed me, and always left me feeling like I could do better. Now, having left it so long, I'd had to devote months to getting into a shape that gave me a realistic chance of even matching that time, and then effectively train my mind to believe that I was capable of pushing just a little bit further. Overall, it had been a massive undertaking. Jo had met me in this final phase. I certainly showed her that I could be passionate and committed, but I imagine she was quietly waiting for this race to be over so that I could spend my time with her rather than constantly training. There was an end date, of course, which would be a release for us both. With this in mind, I knew I couldn't afford to take my foot off the gas. As long as I could look back knowing I'd done my level best, we could move forward together.

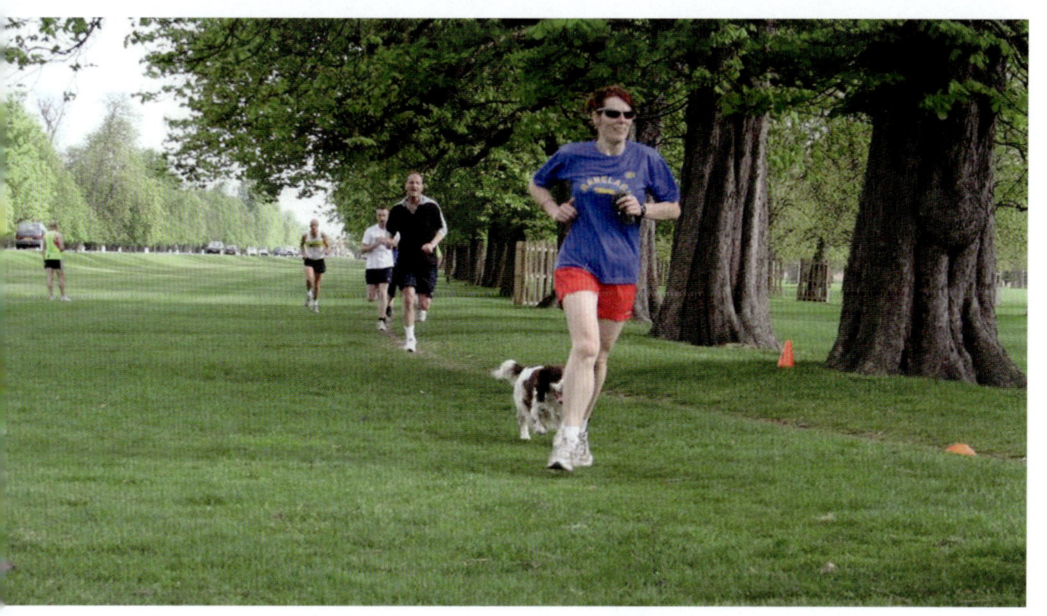

With Timmy in tow, Jo sets the pace at Bushy Park Time Trial in 2006 – when dogs could run off lead.

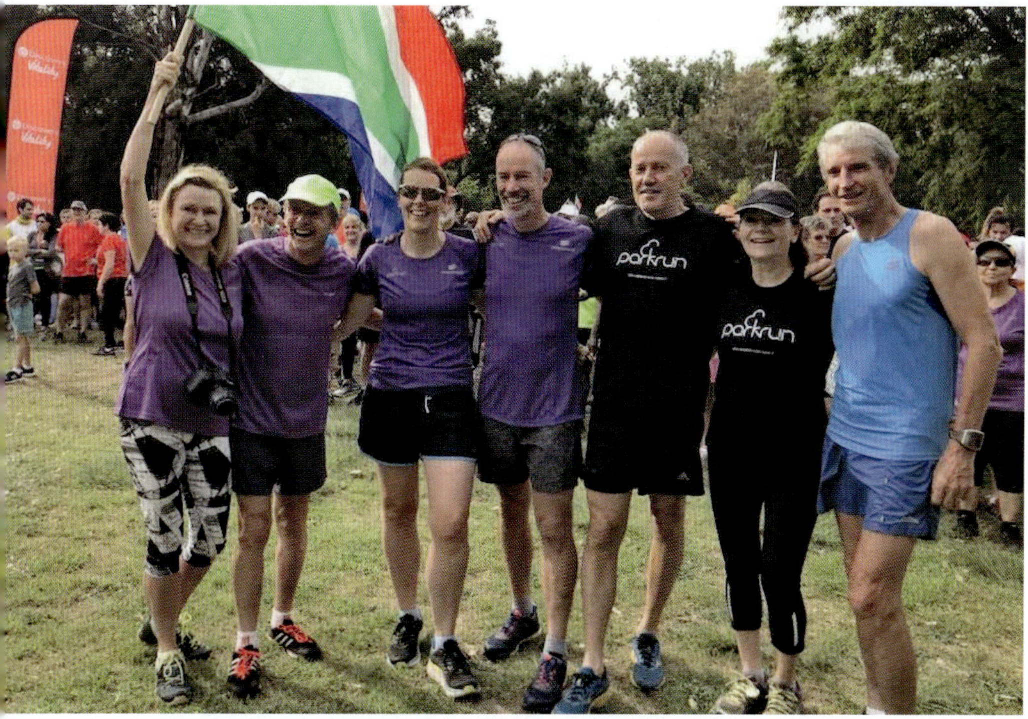

In 2012, Jo and I visited South Africa to celebrate the first anniversary of the country's inaugural *parkrun* at Delta Park in Johannesburg. From left to right: Gill and Bruce Fordyce (who was instrumental in establishing *parkrun* SA) Jo and I in volunteer t-shirts, alongside Noel and Lian DeCharmoy and Brian Chamberlain, another influential figure in my early days as a runner.

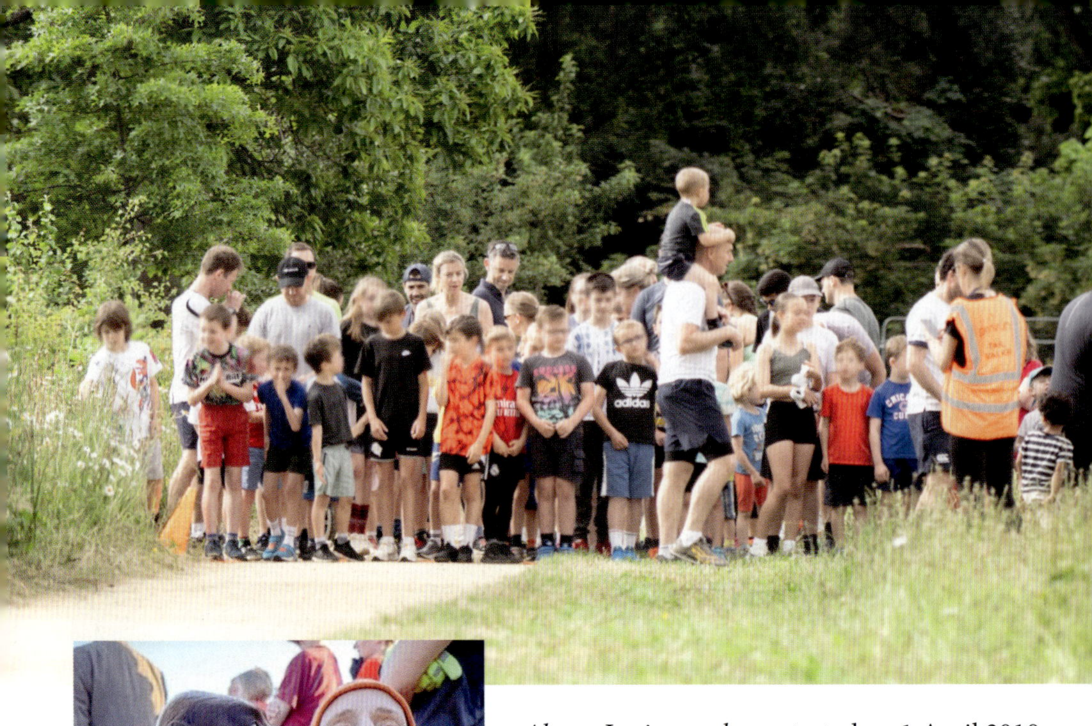

Above: Junior *parkrun* started on 1 April 2010, with the first event held at Bushy Park in London, UK. It has since grown, spreading to multiple locations globally, encouraging kids to get active and enjoy running.

Left: In 2012, when Timmy was ten, Jo and I welcomed another energetic springer spaniel into the family fold. Dotty loved *parkrun*, and could always be relied upon for a finishing face wash.

Right: In April 2019, Futakotamagawa *parkrun* in Japan marked the country's first event. All around the world, the character of each event is shaped by the local community. Here I welcomed everyone alongside the paralympian, Noel Thatcher, who helped to bring *parkrun* to Japan.

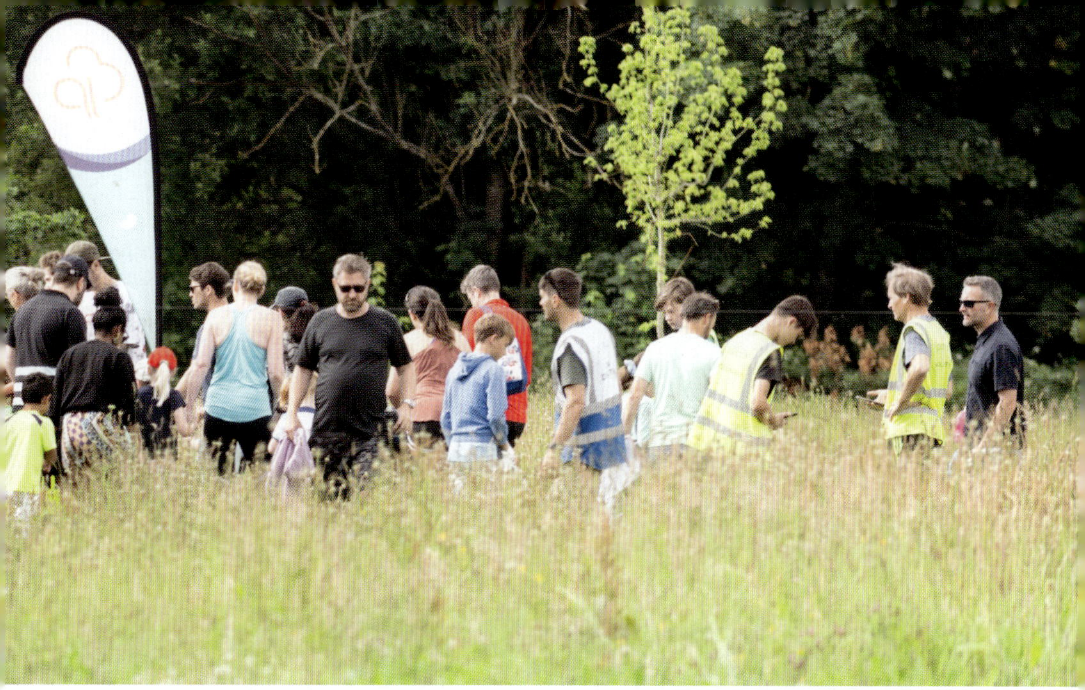

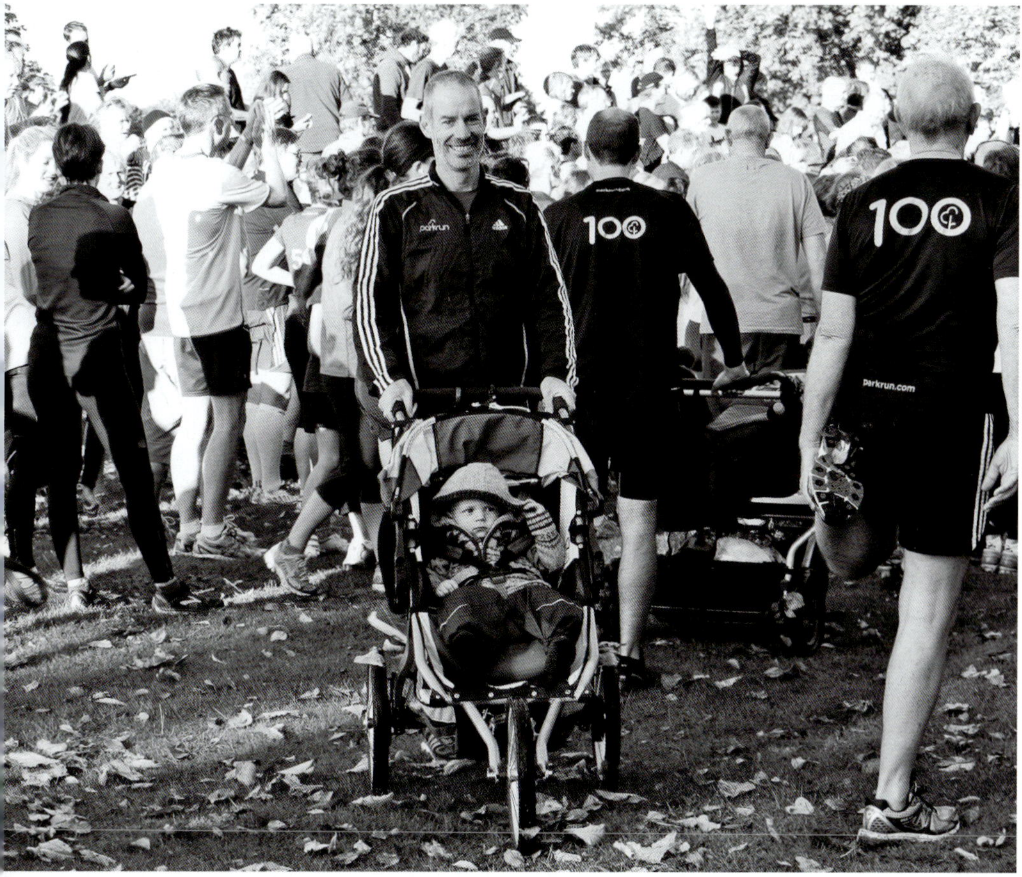

My first Bushy *parkrun* experience as a proud grandfather pushing a buggy.
It was exhausting, but worth it for the memories.

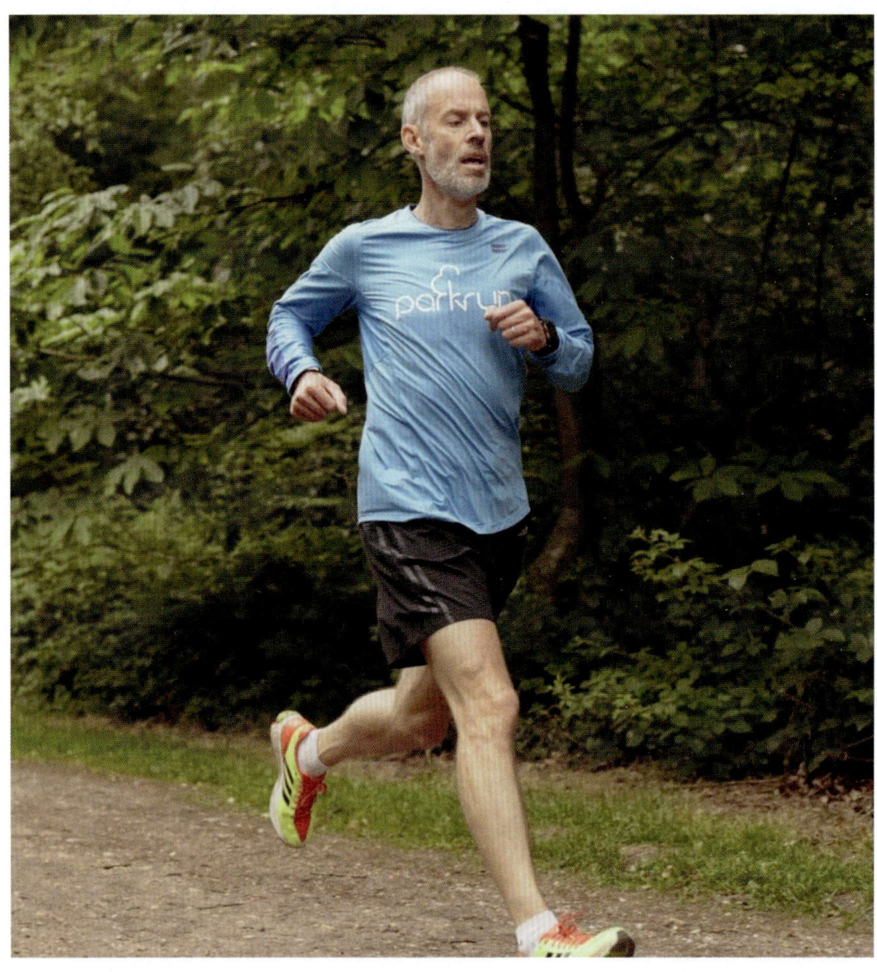

I no longer run in pursuit of a personal best time. When I do lace up my running shoes at *parkrun*, it's all about fun, good company, coffee and cake.

At *parkrun* over the festive period, the Santa hats come out long before 25 December. Jo and I celebrate with friends at a *parkrun* in West Sussex (right). Incognito at Bushy *parkrun* (below).

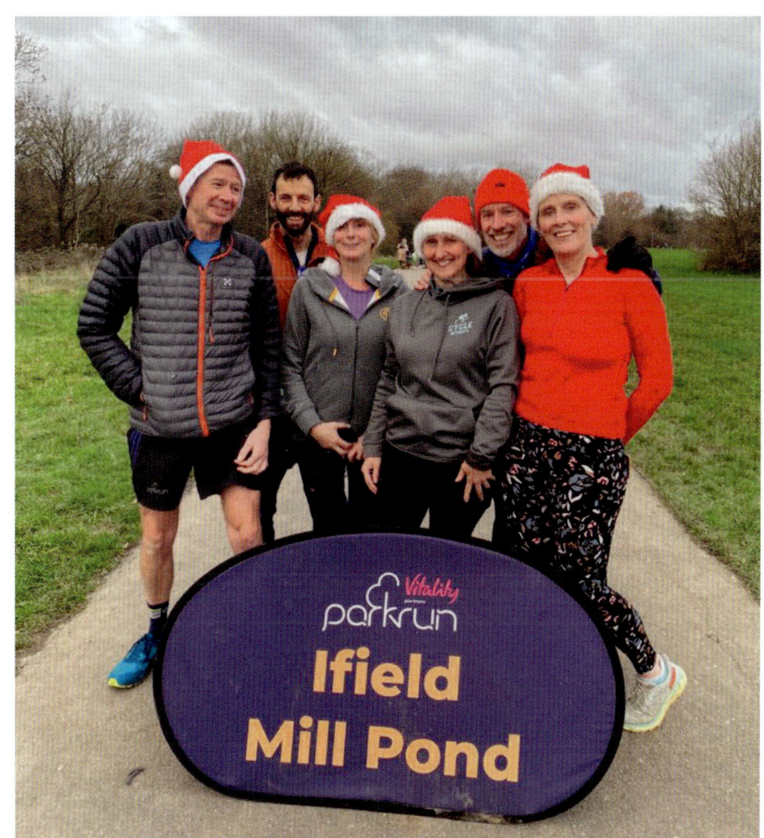

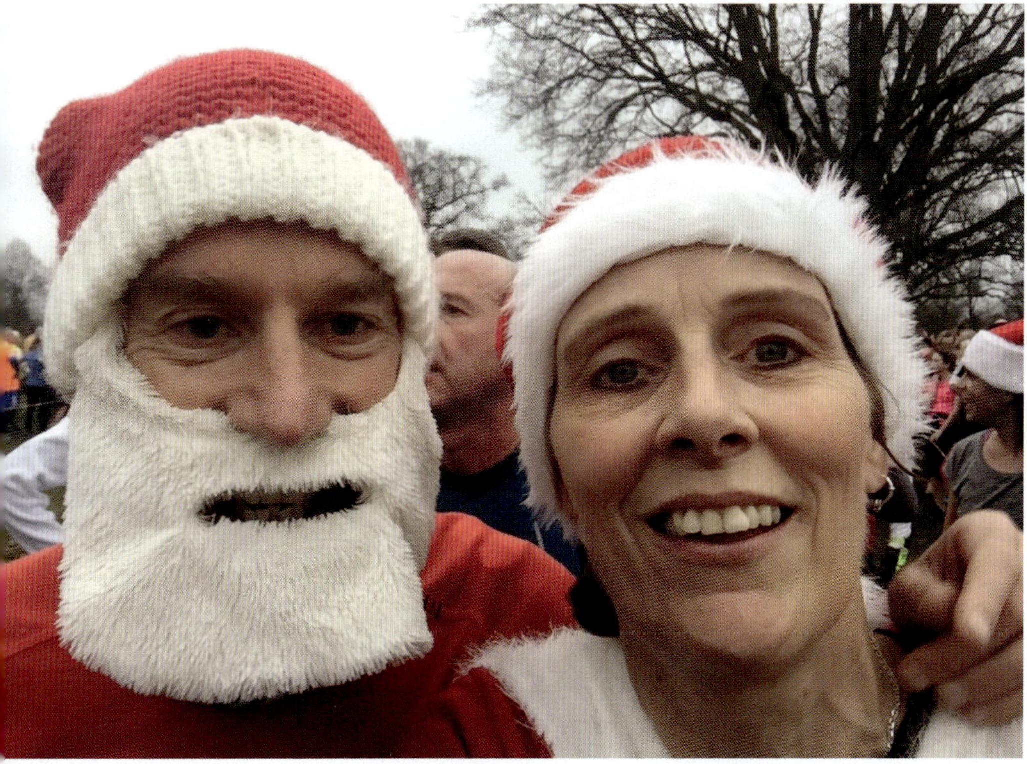

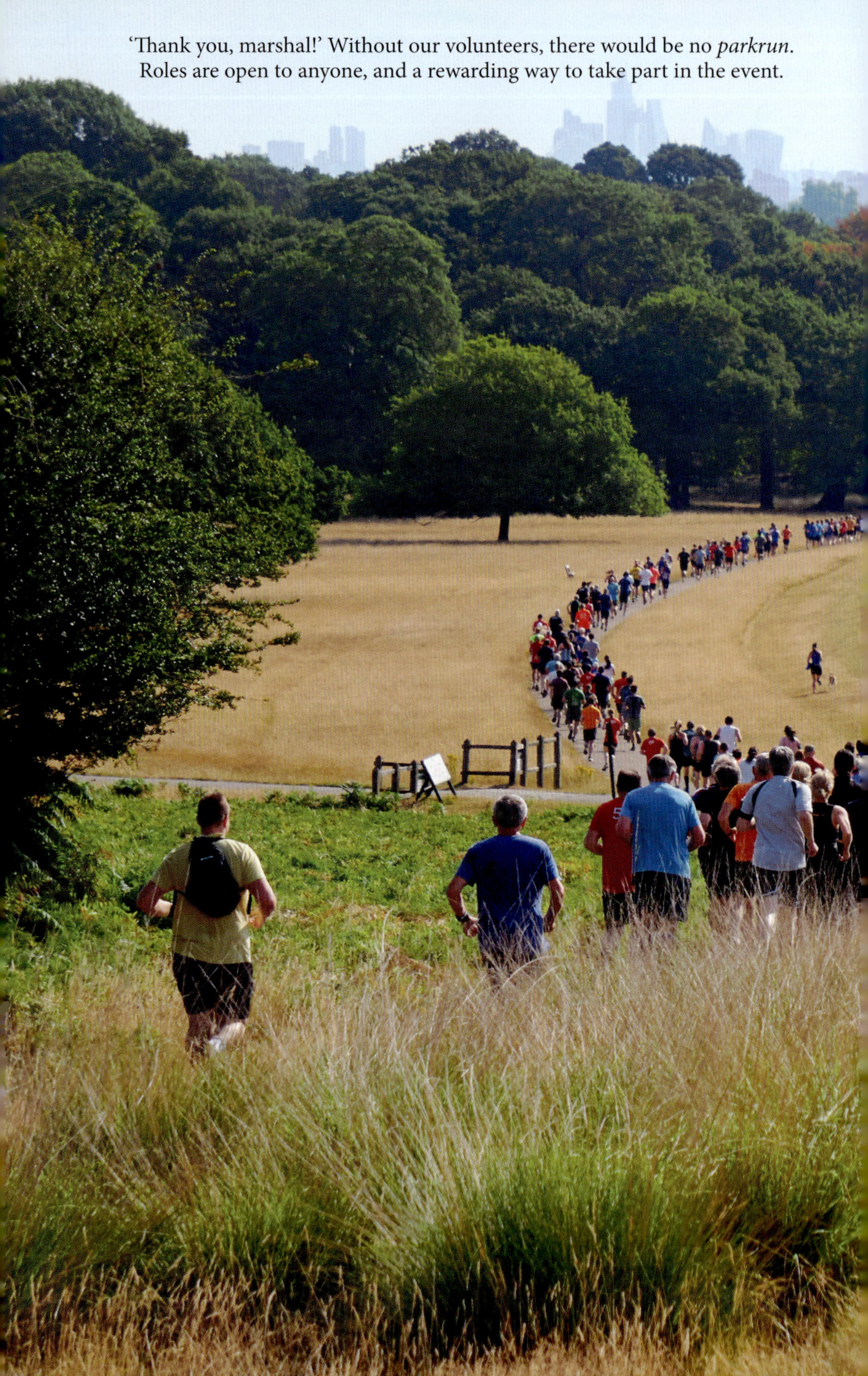

'Thank you, marshal!' Without our volunteers, there would be no *parkrun*. Roles are open to anyone, and a rewarding way to take part in the event.

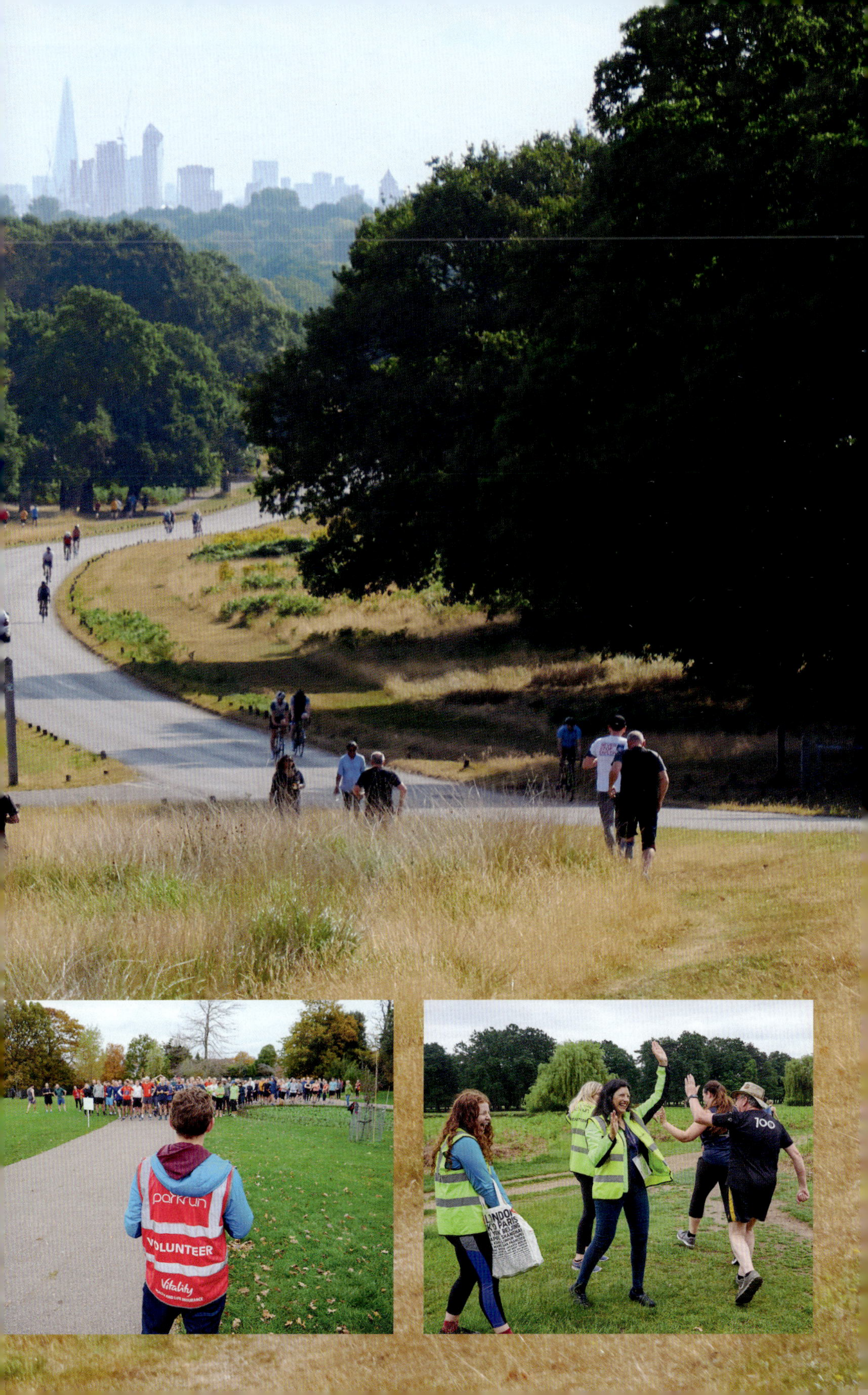
parkrun
VOLUNTEER
Vitality
100

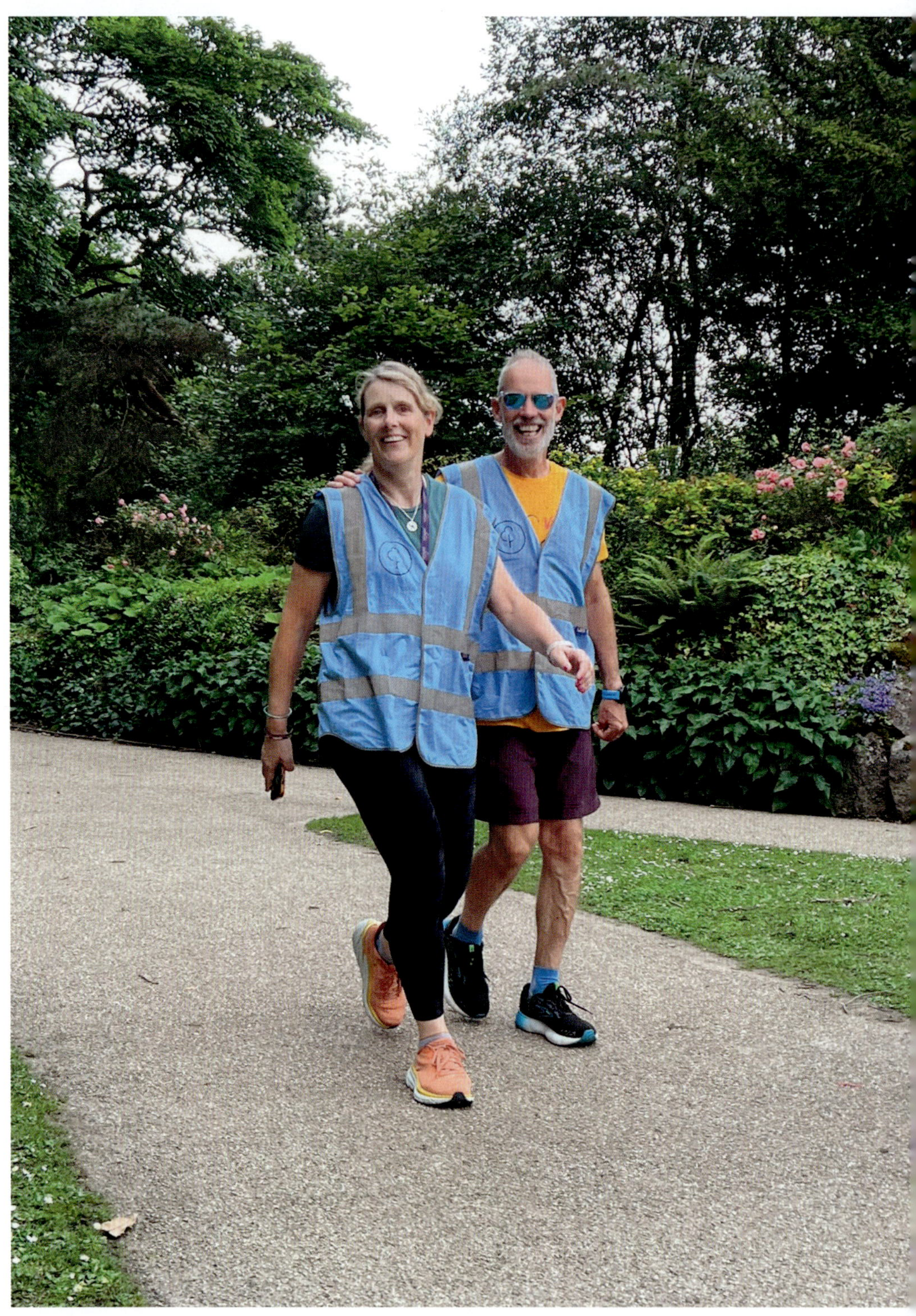

Today, my favourite volunteering role is parkwalker. The aim is to provide encouragement and support to walkers, ensuring they feel welcome and included while highlighting that walking is a valued part of the event. Like any volunteering role at *parkrun*, it's a great opportunity to meet new people and enjoy good conversation.

We were on the home straight now. The race was just the culmination of a longer journey and the chance to end on a high. With the marathon scheduled for April, and spring just around the corner, I had a few final markers to tick off my training list.

First was an annual cross country meet popular with club runners across south-west London. A mob match sounded chaotic and lived up to its name. Five clubs were involved in this season-long face off, which was established in the late 1800s and took the form of a series of one-on-one races between rivals. Participation was key to winning, with the club who fronted the greatest number standing the best chance, but with a weighted scoring system it meant everyone who took part could contribute points. It was so complex that the winning team would often not be known until the last runner had finished, but ultimately the aim was to have fun.

At this fixture, Ranelagh Harriers faced the South London Harriers. It was the turn of our opponents to host the 7.5-mile race, which took place south of the capital on Farthing Down. The looped course took in an elevated expanse of countryside with views of distant skyscrapers before dropping into farmland in the valley. I had brought Tim the dog with me. He didn't contribute points, but added to the general atmosphere of good-natured competition. I had no time in mind. My aim was to stick with the front runners without overstretching myself. If I could finish feeling like I'd completed a workout that would be another tick in the box.

'Are you ready?' I said to my four-legged companion. I could trust Tim to run off lead. We were in a pack, after all, and there was nothing a dog likes more than a group activity. I knew that he would just run alongside me and enjoy the event as much as everyone else. He was also quite a popular team feature, in fact, like a fast-moving mascot that people fussed over at the finish line. 'Let's go!'

It was a bitingly cold Saturday afternoon. My breath turned to puffs of vapour as the initial scramble for position settled down and the pack began to stretch out. As planned, I stayed with the frontrunners in sight for much of the race. The ground was hard and lumpy. Most of my training took place on pavements, and so I had to think about the placement of each footfall. It made a refreshing change, while Tim just bounded effortlessly over divots and ridges without a care in the world.

'Good boy! Keep it up.'

We ran under a boundless blue sky. The chill, crisp air was welcome as my body temperature climbed. When the path peeled into a rolling descent into the valley, it was remarkable how some runners took it in their stride while others appeared to brake. Sensing an advantage to be had, I followed my dog's example and barrelled into the challenge. By the foot of the hill, I had gained a place and turned my attention to the next guy ahead. I felt strong, mindful that I had put in a great deal of training and aware that I could possibly pick up a few extra points for the club. The path took us across a ploughed field. To one side, a marshal in a high-vis tabard stood beside a small gap in the hedgerow. I knew I couldn't catch the runner before he reached the gap. I figured if I could get close then I might be able to make the move stick soon after. Watching us approach, the marshal gestured towards the gap. The runner thanked her in passing and disappeared into the field on the other side. I drew breath to do the same thing, focused solely on giving chase, only for Tim to dart through the gap just a footfall before me. While he made it across my path without making contact with me, as he always did, I instinctively flinched. It was enough for me to catch my footing on a frozen furrow and somersault so spectacularly that I landed on my back in front of a startled marshal.

'I'm fine!' I offered, shot through with adrenalin and embarrassment as I scrambled to my feet. 'All good!'

'Are you sure? That was quite a fall.'

'Thank you for your help!'

I didn't even stop to check for cuts or scrapes. In race mode, I saw it as just a waste of precious seconds that I would have to make up by running that little bit harder.

On the path in the next field, within less than a minute, I had given up on chasing down my quarry. While I tried to shut down any thought that I was injured, my body was telling me otherwise. Something strange was going on with the muscles in my left leg. It felt like they weren't firing properly, while every footfall delivered what felt like a punch to my pelvis. *It can't be serious*, I told myself. *Run it off.*

I held my position in the closing miles, but only because the dog and I had pulled a decent gap ahead of the runners behind us. In truth, I had to slow down considerably because the pain was beginning to bite. I just wanted this race to be over and done with. It was no longer fun, but I didn't want to let down my club. When we finally made it, I limped to one side to sort out a drink for the dog and then assess myself for damage. As nothing hurt as much as it had when I was running, I hoped a day's rest would sort me out.

Waking up the next morning, gritting my teeth as I rolled out of bed, I extended my recovery time to a few days. I hit the painkillers and made a point of stretching in the hope that I was easing out muscle knots and gripes. It was annoying, but running accidents happened. By now, my back had started aching. It felt stiff, as did my bad leg. I put it down to inflammation and bruising and just focused on work and family. By midweek, I set out for a gentle run to the park. I was aware that I might be sore. I just hadn't anticipated that I'd be grimacing as soon I put one foot in front of the other. I could run but it hurt. By rights, I should have rested. As a runner with a goal, however, I hadn't reached that point of acceptance. I had a plan and needed to see it through. Having come this far, I couldn't let a little discomfort defeat me.

So, despite the fact that it caused me pain, I pressed on with my running programme. I still monitored my pace and gritted my teeth to maintain it. On my first run with Duncan Gaskell, he recognized that something was wrong from the moment we set off.

'I can put you in touch with a top physio,' he suggested, speaking as a sports agent as much as a friend, but I remained convinced that I could run it off.

'It'll pass,' I said, picking up the pace a little as if to prove it.

In the days that followed, I sensed myself growing anxious about my form. I continued to train. It's just my plan didn't cater for a runner in pain. It compromised everything from my rhythm and pace, steadily disrupting my focus. My blinkers were on, however. I had the London Marathon in my sights and wasn't prepared to let anything get in the way. As part of the last stage of my preparations, I had entered a couple of shorter, punchier races to help measure and assess my progress. Ignoring what my body was trying to tell me, I ran a local 10K in a personal best of just under 33 minutes. It took me out of my comfort zone, but I had become accustomed to that feeling and learned to just hold on. Back home, I explored my time and pace data, as well as taking attrition into account, to calculate that I was still on course to meet my marathon target. Then, in complete denial about the state I was in, I completed the Windsor Half Marathon in 1 hour and 15 minutes. As a measure of the effort I put into it, ignoring how much it hurt, I finished in tenth place. Like the earlier 10K, if I used it as a measure of what I could achieve in a full marathon then my time was consistent with the same outcome. Over double the distance, if everything went to plan, I could hope to run 26.2 miles in under two and half hours.

At home, I tried to downplay how much everything hurt. I just let myself down on that front by complaining about it all the time.

'Can you defer the place to next year?' Jo asked.

In my mind, it wasn't an option. Even if the regulations allowed it, I knew that skipping a year would only eat me up. The London Marathon had moved in on my life. If I could just run it according to my prediction then I could effectively return to the family having got it out of my system.

By mid-March, just one remaining race stood between

me and the London Marathon. The Bath Half Marathon was intended to be my final push. If I could repeat the same finishing time I had chalked up in Windsor, or even improve on it slightly, it would give me a shot of confidence that could take me far the following month. Given how much it had hurt on my last outing, however, I was in two minds about running at all. I was even starting to walk with a limp to minimize the pain.

I left it to the last minute to make a decision. Inevitably, I decided to race. Friends from the club had also entered, and so I even offered to drive.

Since my fall, every time I set off on a run, I quietly hoped for a miracle. I yearned to take a step and find all pain had gone. Instead, as the Bath Half Marathon got underway, I knew that I would be in for a rough time. In a way, it spurred me on. The quicker I ran, I resolved, the sooner I could put myself out of my misery. This time, in a crowded race around the city's streets, I found myself negotiating a lot of pavements. About halfway round, those small steps up and down from the kerb became something I learned to dread. The jolt of pain took my breath away. It even led to my limp making an appearance as I counted down the miles to the finish line. I felt physically fit. The problem was several moving parts appeared to be seizing up. With my eyes on my watch, and then the timer on the finishing gantry, I pressed myself over the line two minutes quicker than I had ever run a half marathon before. I should have been elated, but by then only one race mattered to me.

Staggering to a halt, I did the maths in my mind. Despite the pain and effort it had taken, I was still just within my target window for the marathon.

With the medal around my shoulders, and a cup of water in hand, I took myself to a patch of grass where finishers were sprawled and sat down. As I did so, the abrupt spasm in my back told me that I wouldn't be getting up in a hurry. I tried to relax in the hope that the spasm would ease. Instead it responded by twisting and tightening. I didn't want to make a scene, despite the pain, but when I spotted one of my friends from the club finishing his race I waved him over with some urgency.

'I'm in trouble,' I said, which was probably obvious given my contorted position. 'Can you help me to the car?'

My friend stood over me, contemplating what I'd just said.

'Am I insured to drive?' he asked. 'There's no way you can get behind the wheel.'

Despite my protest that it would loosen off, and with the assistance of another club runner who had travelled with us, I found I couldn't even settle in the passenger seat. Whatever I had done to myself in a mob match fall was now screaming at me for attention. All I could do was hand over the car key and lie across the back seat for the journey home. I couldn't even think about what it meant for my training plan that week. I was in agony.

Having politely brushed off Duncan's offer to put me in touch with a physio, I returned home to make an appointment at the earliest opportunity. A few days later, after he had assessed me, I waited for him to finish typing up my notes. As he had also drawn the full story from me about how I'd been running through pain in the hope that it would magically disappear, I felt like an idiot. While it was a relief to be in professional care at last, I knew that I only had myself to blame for whatever he had to tell me. My stubbornness had led me to ignore all the warning signs. Now I was set to pay the price.

'There is no easy fix here.' The physio turned from his screen to face me. As I listened to him reel off the list of injuries I was carrying, I defaulted to the mindset I'd developed growing up. Faced with someone in a position of authority, I could have no say in the outcome. Whatever his diagnosis, I would simply have to go along with it. 'Paul, I'm afraid running is out of the question.'

'So, like a week?' I asked, with April's marathon in mind. 'A *month*?'

'We're talking years,' said the physio, and from that moment on I stopped listening as he sought to soften the diagnosis with talk of the long rehabilitation programme I faced.

19

ONE SMALL STEP

I had mixed emotions about that year's London Marathon. On the one hand I was keen to support friends and club mates who were running. On the other, sidelined from an activity that I loved, I sensed a return of that bleak feeling I had carried through my life from the children's home to the boarding house and the aftermath of my marriage. It would always be there, I realized, lurking in the background. It was just that running held it at bay and even brought light into my life in the form of Jo and a new shape to my family that I adored.

Once the shock and disbelief subsided, having learned that my goal had gone, I had to face up to the wider consequences. It was one thing to come to terms with the fact that all my training efforts had amounted to nothing, but quite another to realize that even the simple act of running was no longer available to me. I had torn my abdominal muscles, my glutes and a hamstring. As everything was connected, any attempt to run just led to stresses, strain, pain and a cascade effect in terms of the problems I faced. While a combination of rest and physiotherapy had eased my back issues, I was still in a great deal of pain. Even walking was difficult, and I found myself limping around at home. Even if I could find a job, I brooded to myself in those first weeks until the pain became more manageable, I wasn't sure that I would be physically capable of holding it down. Feeling low, I reverted to my old ways of not talking about how I was feeling. People didn't want to hear me moaning, I decided. So, I shut it away.

The physio had given me a raft of exercises. He had also been realistic about the timeframe for my recovery. Frankly, I couldn't process that it would be at least eighteen months before I could even think about a short, gentle jog. I had all but written off a return to my previous form. Even if I could overcome the damage I had done to myself, I couldn't see any chance that I would be able to revive my running dream. I would be older for one thing, with my best years behind me. I felt like I had come tantalizingly close to running a sub two-and-a-half-hour marathon. I'd followed the training plan religiously, and all the signs were there to suggest I was on course to break that barrier. For so long, that finishing time had meant everything to me. Now it had gone, and I was left with a dream that suddenly seemed quite meaningless. As I stewed on things while hobbling around, I came to see it as nothing more than an arbitrary number. There was no value to it. Running a sub 2.30 marathon didn't make the world a better place. And even if I had achieved my goal, I realized, chances are I would have only set my sights on a quicker time.

With this enforced distance from something that had consumed me, I recognized what it was that I missed more than anything else. It wasn't the chance to chase a time. It was the bonds I made with people through running that helped me to feel like I belonged. That was the true value at the heart of this activity that I loved. Running had given me that social connection I craved in growing up. As the days grew warmer and brighter with the approach of summer, I really missed the sense of joy that came from running with my friends. Without it, I felt as if I was back on the same sidelines I had occupied as a kid. This time, I wasn't wary about getting involved. I just couldn't run.

'Why don't you join them when they've finished?' Jo suggested in a bid to lift my spirits.

Even though I didn't put it into words, she knew how much I missed the group run every week. As everyone capped off the evening with a drink in the pub next door to the clubhouse, it seemed like a good idea. I didn't like feeling sorry for myself, after all. I was also sensitive to the fact that Jo had picked up on it. The last thing I wanted to do was drag her down with me. Given that she wouldn't be the only one to register me moping, or silently willing the phone to ring with good news in my search for work, I knew that it would be better for everyone if I was out of the house.

Before my injury, I considered the Tuesday evening group session to be the highlight of my running week.

My training could be solitary, and this was an opportunity to be social. Even if I chose to go out with a faster lot, with little opportunity for chat, that all changed after we regrouped in the pub with refreshments in hand. That was something I could still participate in, I reminded myself on settling into a corner table at the pub that evening. I had arrived early enough to see the groups as they set off. Some roamed across the park as the sun set. Others cast long shadows as they trotted along the pavements and side roads. I was so pleased to see them all and looked forward to catching up once they were done.

Nursing a beer on my own, and then another just to kill the next hour, I couldn't help but register how much those sessions meant to me.

By the time the first runners entered, I had been looking at the clock on the wall so frequently that time appeared to be standing still. They were no later than usual, but by then I had grown restless in my own company. I was also a couple of pints into the evening. So, when the table I had reserved started filling with runners, I was primed for a good time. As I had hoped, the chatter flowed. It's just everything was pinned to that evening's group sessions. Bathed in a post-run glow, people either picked up on topics they'd already started or relived moments they'd shared together. I tried to find a way to join in with the conversation, but nothing opened up for me. All I could do was listen, feeling behind on the chat but ahead on the drinks, and that really wasn't me.

As a non-runner, the Tuesday evening group just wasn't

the same. After persevering for a few more dispiriting weeks, I decided to stay at home.

I had tripped up during a training run. Months later, it felt like I was still falling. Without running in my life, I'd lost the means of keeping both my mind and body in shape. For some time, I worked hard to be positive about the situation. I reminded myself that other pursuits were available, like swimming and cycling, but I couldn't shake off the feeling that giving up running had also cost me a social life. Feeling sidelined once again, that sense of unfairness began to register in my mind as it had throughout my childhood.

Since the accident, I found the search for work had taken on a new meaning. I wasn't just looking for employment, I realized, but also a purpose. All I could do was keep backing myself, but that was hard when I had no means of mentally resetting and recharging as I once had as a runner. Although I still couldn't walk without a slight limp, there had to be a way to stay involved with running and the people who shared my passion for it.

I thought back to my early years as a runner in South Africa. People grouped together either casually or in clubs, and in Johannesburg that had created a vibrant running scene. In particular, I had really enjoyed the time trial culture. I liked the way that the clubs worked together to offer runners across the city a chance to measure their performance on a regular basis. It was an informal, friendly arrangement and essentially an excuse during the weekday evenings for people to get together and do the thing they loved. Above all, it introduced me to runners I wouldn't otherwise have met, and widened my circle of friends.

Since moving to the UK from South Africa, I had always been struck by the cultural difference. Running was just as popular here, but clubs tended to keep to themselves outside of organized races. Some put on time trials, but only as an occasional event and in general just for their members. I was also aware that many runners in my adopted country weren't even associated with a club. It was often seen as a solitary activity, whereas I had grown up in a country that went wild for the likes of Comrades. There, running was considered to be more of a communal event.

With this in mind, I wondered whether maybe I could create something that would give me a role in a world that I loved while also bringing people together. Whatever that looked like, I was clear that it shouldn't just be for elite runners. I wanted it to bring out the best in everyone. It had to be open to all abilities.

Throughout that early summer, I kept coming back to my idea. If I could pitch my event as a social activity, perhaps it would encourage runners not just from clubs but also those outside them. And if it appealed to people who didn't consider themselves to be competitive runners, I would be sharing my enthusiasm for something that I knew from personal experience could become a lifesaver.

With nothing but dead ends in my search for work, I found this personal project of mine at least helped to keep my anxieties at bay. It also gave me that valuable sense of purpose. I knew that I would make it happen, but I was also in no rush because I wanted to do it properly. When I shared my proposal with Jo, her first question about it was both simple and direct.

'Why?' she asked. 'You might get a few people to come along, but what's in it for you?'

I smiled in response. Jo had effectively provided the answer.

'It could be good,' I said eventually. 'For everyone.'

As the plan for my own take on a time trial evolved in my mind, I found myself talking to Jo about it at length. She was nothing but supportive. Even though our relationship was still young, she recognized what was behind my determination to make it happen. Jo knew how much running meant to me, and if this venture helped me to lift my spirits then she knew that could only benefit us both.

'Just keep it simple,' she advised early on, and I took that to heart

As well as being easy to understand, I wanted no obstacles that could deter people from taking part. As I made notes and laid down the foundations for a process to make it happen, the challenges started to take shape. In Johannesburg during the eighties, it had always been possible to find a time trial at least once a fortnight somewhere in the city. There was no formal calendar. We'd just had to rely on club newsletters or word of mouth. This seemed to me like a barrier to entry. If people had to make an effort to find out when and where my event was happening, it could only prevent some from showing up. It had to be at the same time and place on a regular basis. This wasn't something I saw as a one-off or a series that would come to an end if my running legs ever returned to me. It needed to become a permanent feature of the landscape without any need for people to check if, when and where it was taking place.

In opening it up to everyone, I wasn't proposing a race. It would be a regular timed run that allowed anyone who came along to get whatever they wanted from it. My time trial could be used as a way for people to assess their fitness or measure training progress, because I would be on hand with my stopwatch. Everybody would get a time and a position, but there would be no winners or losers. Whatever personal aims anyone brought to the start line, it all came down to a shared love of running. I just had to work out how to make it all happen.

Some decisions were easier for me to make than others. High up on my list was the fact that my time trial should be free. There would be no charge of any kind. A local running event was hardly going to be a get-rich-quick scheme, but more importantly the only thing I wanted to make from the venture was friends. By also doing away with conventional running club membership requirements and any kind of entry fee or qualification, I just hoped to appeal to as many people as possible.

In South Africa, some time trials could extend to 10K. Much depended on the course a club could cobble together, either as an out-and-back or a loop so it started and finished in the same place for convenience. As much as I enjoyed running a longer time trial, it could catch out seasoned runners if they went out too hot.

For my event, I settled on 5K as a suitable distance for two reasons. Firstly, it seemed accessible to everyone. Secondly, it wouldn't take up too much time, not just mine but also anyone who showed up. People led busy lives, after all. For a while, I toyed with locating the event in Richmond Park. It was only a mile or so from my house in Twickenham, with a prominent gateway that could serve as an easily identifiable meeting point. In the end, Bushy Park won out because it was even closer to where I lived. I intended to be in and out, and then ultimately back home with minimal disruption.

I knew it had to be a weekend event. That would be most convenient to people, I thought, including me. The question was when. Sundays were traditionally reserved for club meets and races, which meant Saturday was the obvious choice to maximize appeal. An afternoon event would appeal to those who enjoyed a lie-in after the working week. The way I saw it, however, a later start risked losing people to the demands of the day. For me, the early morning was a quiet period before everyone drifted into other things.

As for the start time, my initial idea was subject to revision by a loose group of friends. Even though I'd stopped joining the Harriers in the pub after their Tuesday run because it reminded me of what I was missing, Jo and I still went out for drinks occasionally with club members we knew from Ranelagh and also the Stragglers. Over the summer months, they got to know about my project and would question me with interest about how it was shaping up. Towards the autumn of 2004, having set a starting date in order to focus my efforts, I found myself with an informal sounding board I could trust.

'Eight o'clock seems good to me,' I proposed when the subject arose. 'Bright and early.'

Around the table, people looked at me as if I'd just suggested I couldn't afford to pay for my round.

'Paul, you're not in South Africa now.' Andrew Lane, a veteran Stragglers runner, appeared to be speaking for everyone. 'It hardly gets too hot to run here. It's too early. If you want people to show up, make it nine.'

Prompted by the nods of approval, I scrubbed out the time I had written in my notebook.

'Tell everyone what it's called,' Duncan Gaskell spoke up as I jotted down the new time. I looked across the table to find him grinning mischievously. 'Go on.'

Setting down my pen, I held up my hands as if to frame the proposed name.

'Bushy Park Time Trial.' While I knew my savvy sports agent friend had his doubts about the name, I hadn't expected such complete silence. Nor did I think everyone would respond by looking at the table or reaching awkwardly for their drinks. 'It does what it says on the tin,' I reasoned, as if that might help to sell it. Having put so much effort into working on the format, and identifying the procedures that would allow me to make it happen, I felt that I was about to introduce an event in the local running calendar that was accessible to all if nothing else. 'Beginning next Saturday . . . at nine o'clock.'

'What if nobody shows up?'

Jim Desmond had been very good at challenging the working parts of my proposal. He could be direct, but I valued his input.

'I'll still be there,' I said. 'At the same time every week.'

'For how long?' he asked.

I glanced at Jo. Already wise to my plan, she had

responded with the same raised eyebrows as Jim, Duncan and the rest of my friends around the table when I answered him.

'For ever,' I said, as if anyone even needed to ask.

PART THREE

Bushy Park, Richmond, south-west London
Saturday, 4 October 2004
9.00 a.m.

'Go!'

As I start the first Bushy Park Time Trial, Jo stands across from me and offers words of encouragement to the runners.

'Good luck,' she says, watching them stream between us. 'Enjoy it.'

In the last hour, a blustery breeze has picked up across the park. It's a little chilly and so I imagine everyone who has shown up must be glad to be on their way. Together, we watch the last participant hop onto the grass alongside the short road to the park's fountain feature. Jo remarks that it's all gone to plan so far.

'We've only just begun,' I say.

I watch the small knot of runners begin to loosen as everyone finds their pace. When they pick up the path that takes them out towards the park's perimeter, I'm heartened to hear some chatter from some and even laughter. Alongside Jo, a couple of friends have come along to help out. Robin is here because his wife is one of the runners, while Alan from Ranelagh Harriers is the keeper of the club's stopwatch. It's no ordinary device, and I've asked to borrow it so I can make full use of the special features. Having brought it along for me, Alan even offered to stay and lend a hand. I'm really grateful to them all for their support.

'At least it wasn't hard to get everyone in shot,' Robin jokes with Alan, who had borrowed my digital camera to take photographs.

By now, the runners are well on their way. In my brief before the start, I had stressed that it wasn't a competition. People could run as hard as they liked, and use the opportunity to assess their fitness, but ultimately it was intended as a bit of fun for everyone. I just hope I'm not alone in believing that would strike a chord.

'Paul . . .'

It's Jo who draws my attention from the little screen.

'What's up?'

As Alan previews the photographs he's taken, and Robin peers over his shoulder, I find her looking at me reassuringly.

'Everything is going to be OK.'

We walk the short distance to the finishing line, marked by the fourth tree along beside the stream as determined by my adventures with the trundle wheel. On the way, I fall in with the last person who has joined me this morning. As soon as Duncan Gaskell arrived, having spent the last few weeks stress-testing my idea as I developed it, I read his presence as a quiet nod of approval.

'You can be sure that the club will be up to speed by next

week,' he says with a grin, nodding at our two friends from Ranelagh. I know that Robin and Alan are here because they're kind and also interested. It isn't lost on me, however, that others at the club will press them for details of the event.

'Let's hope it's all positive,' I say.

While nobody has objected to my time trial, I have encountered some resistance from the running community. In a way I expected it. As I talked it through with my friends in the pub, a view had taken shape that this was something new that could potentially upset the way of things. If too many club members took up the opportunity to run for free with me on Saturdays, some said, it could deter them from paying to enter a race on Sundays. The way I see things, there is room for everything and also everyone – which is why I have wanted to make this an independent venture. Most importantly to me, I'm not just here for club runners. I'm so determined that people don't mistake this for a race that I have two identical prizes to hand out. One for the first runner to cross the line and the other for the last.

As for finishing times and positions, which I want to record to create a picture of the event, I've put together a system that is being road-tested for the first time. In a short while from now, with a thumb click as each runner finishes, I'll use the club's fancy stopwatch in my hand to assign a time to each position. It'll then spool out a list like a shopping receipt that will help me to compile the results. When it comes to catching and recording names, I have resorted to a very basic measure. Having crossed the finish line, each runner will collect a steel washer from Jo. She's clutching a string of fifty on a loop of wire. Each washer is stamped with a number to denote a finishing position, and looks about as amateur as it sounds because I made them myself.

Earlier in the week, I had visited a hardware shop to purchase a number-punching kit and hammer along with the washers. Working outside on my patio, I then set about individually imprinting digits into the rim of each one. I knew that I was producing an ambitious amount, and it took a while to complete on reaching double figures. In some ways it just helped me stay true to my belief that if I kept showing up at the same place in the park at nine o'clock every Saturday morning then more people would come. Annoyingly, I also managed to crack a flagstone in the process of stamping each washer. I told myself it was a small price to pay should I have to cater for a turnout one weekend beyond my wildest dreams.

Just under nineteen minutes after they set off, the first two runners wheel into view at the far end of the tree funnel. Both are neck and neck, but clearly have the same outcome in mind. With the space of one tree to go, Chris Owens and Matthew Morgan clasp hands to cross the line. It's a finish marked by laughter and cheers, along with jokes about having to tear in half the prize I present them. The ten-pound gift vouchers have been kindly donated by Sweatshop, a local running store who committed to providing one weekly prize. In my mind, the joint finish sums up the spirit of my event. It's been fun, and not just for the runners.

'Everyone's a winner,' says Jo as yet more finishers file past her to collect their hand-numbered finishing washer and then gather in the clearing beyond the next tree to recover their breath. Among them is my friend from the Stragglers, Andrew Lane, who is responsible for earning everyone here an extra

hour in bed this morning, as well as Ranelagh runners including Julie Drummond whose husband was clapping everyone in. As the number of finishers grows, people begin to exchange a few words with each other about the experience they've just shared. By the time I click through the final two runners, who also cross the line together, everyone is chatting away in the afterglow of an event that feels to me like it might have legs.

'When you're ready,' I say to everyone, gesturing at my car that I've parked in a space on the other side of the stream and left with the boot open, 'write down your finishing position, name and email address on a clipboard I've left out for you and then drop your washer into the cup beside it. I'll email you the results as soon as I've processed them.'

As people begin to drift back to the car park, several make a point of thanking me, Jo, Alan, Robin and Duncan for making the event happen.

'I'll be back,' I hear someone say, which is great to hear but reminds me that this first run of the Bushy Park Time Trial isn't over yet. In my view, the best bit has yet to come.

'One more thing,' I call out. 'We're going to the cafe now for coffee and cake. If anyone would like to join us, I'd be delighted . . .'

20

SPREAD THE WORD

Thirteen people took part in my first time trial at Bushy Park. One week later, on Saturday at nine o'clock, fourteen set off from the start line in the car park.

As I started the stopwatch for the second event, the numbers didn't concern me. I was happy that one more person had come along, but what really mattered was the experience. Once again, people seemed to enjoy themselves, and I counted myself among them.

Throughout the week in between, I had found myself looking forward to the next time trial. I dwelled on what I could do to improve a system that allowed anyone to show up and receive a recorded time and position. In a bid to be efficient, I decided that I should bring a list to each event of all the people who had ever taken part in a time trial. So, rather than writing down their name and email address afresh on the clipboard in the boot of my car, return participants could just find their entry and add their position. That made life easier for them, even if it would mean extra work for me in the week as I updated the database with the details of any first-timers who had scribbled in their details the previous weekend.

Throughout, my aim was to keep things as straightforward as possible. Happily, everyone had picked up on the process. They provided me with the information that I needed after finishing, and even dropped their washers into the pot I'd left out for them. After we'd visited the coffee shop near the park, occupying a couple of tables on the second floor, I headed home to start work in front of my computer. As a runner, I had set out to make the time trial as accessible as possible to all. As a computer systems specialist, I aimed to do the same thing with the results. I'd already devised a simple programme that allowed me to collate all the data I had gathered. It also allowed me to send out the results to all the participants by email, along with a covering note reminding everyone that I'd be there every Saturday, before joining Jo to get on with the rest of our weekend.

'Success?' she had asked as I appeared downstairs.

For me, on the sidelines due to injury, the morning had been a second chance to spend time with people who shared my passion for running. That had to be better than drifting around at home feeling washed-up and forgotten. It gave me the purpose I needed, drew me out of the house and allowed me to hang out with Jo and our friends. That everyone seemed to get something from the experience just strengthened my belief that it had to be worthwhile. At the same time, this wasn't about a short series of informal runs. If I was to define it as a success in my mind then first people had to recognize that Bushy Park Time Trial had become a concrete weekly fixture in the running calendar.

'It's a start,' I had said, before we set out to make the most of the day.

At the third event, the number of people who joined me in the car park just before nine o'clock dropped to eleven. It made no odds to me. A few runners from Ranelagh were shaping up to become regulars, but even with the smaller group it still felt like I was meeting new people every week. I took that as a positive sign. Apart from the flyers I had distributed for the first time trial, I was relying on participants to spread the word. Everyone seemed to leave fired up by the experience, and so I hoped that perhaps they would mention it to others over the course of the week. If it took a month, a year or a decade, I knew that the only way to make the time trial something that resonated was to stay true to my promise and just be there every week at the same time and place.

Given that I intended to make this a permanent feature of the park, I had to make sure that I could manage it on my own. It was one thing for me to pledge to show up every Saturday morning for runners, but I didn't expect anyone to make the same commitment just to help me out. Even so, at each time trial there would always be a few people who offered to support me. It wasn't just Jo or Duncan. Sometimes a partner or friend of a runner would offer to direct participants off the path towards the finish or take over the clipboard entry duties to make life easier for everyone. As well as being so thankful for their support,

I particularly enjoyed the chat we shared together once the time trial was underway and we were left to wait for the runners to come full circle.

We were doing something for others, but the sense of togetherness left me thinking that helping out could be just as rewarding as taking part in the run itself.

On the fourth Saturday, I was prepared to see fewer than ten people. Even if nobody joined me, there was always the following week. Happily, I set off twenty runners around the course that morning, and then crossed to the finish line with my generous helpers and a spring in my step.

'It's a lovely morning,' I said, and though I was zipped up in my jacket the air felt crisp rather than cold.

'It always is,' observed the partner of one of the runners. 'Ever since you started this, it's never rained first thing on a Saturday.'

I glanced across at her to register the point. She was right. We'd had some poor weather on moving from October into November. The temperature had dropped, and in keeping with the season the ground off the pathways was becoming soft underfoot. Even so, whenever I started the stopwatch, the sun was always shining.

By nature, I am not a superstitious person. I'd encountered enough challenges in life to know that luck played no role one way or the other. I joked that divine intervention kept the rain at bay to encourage more people to join us. In reality, it seemed to me that those who came were drawn in part by the communal spirit of the event. Ultimately, it relied on participants recognizing that it was about more than just a free, weekly, timed run and spread the word.

Whatever the weather when I opened the curtains on a Saturday morning, my role was to guarantee the opportunity for people to find out for themselves by making my way to the park.

Faced with the reality of unemployment in middle age, grinding out applications for tech-sector roles in a competitive market, I had plenty of time to reflect on what I had started here. It was nothing fancy, but it meant a lot to me and seemed to make an impression on others, too. I realized that I could have just as easily done nothing about the idea when it came to me. It was only by acting on it that I had made something happen. With this in mind, and with my savings running out, I began to wonder whether I should review my approach to job hunting. It seemed to me that I was seeking employment in the tech sector at a time when companies were shedding jobs and commissioning contractors. While working to get things up and running at Bushy Park, I'd flirted with the idea of starting a consultancy. In doing so, I came to realize, I would be creating a career opportunity for myself. Just as I had with the time trial, it would be a chance to grow a venture from scratch and see where it might take me.

Later that autumn, having reinvented myself as a consultant in software system architecture – a fancy way of saying an expert for hire on a project-by-project basis – I secured work at last. When Vodafone commissioned me in an area of telecommunications where I felt that I could shine, I practically floated into their Berkshire headquarters. Having been through such a bleak time, it seemed to me that the time trial had restored the sense that I still had something to offer. It was a different way of working, of course, trading job security for flexibility, but having been through so much it felt like I was on solid ground at last. With a stable relationship back home, and a means of staying involved with the running world, I approached the end of 2004 determined not to let any of it slip through my fingers.

That year, Christmas Day fell on a Saturday. In the preceding weeks, usually at the end of the run, people would enquire if I planned to take a festive break from my weekly post in the park. The time trial was ticking along, attracting some two dozen participants from one event to the next. The numbers were manageable, but no measure of the enthusiasm, and that was the only thing I registered.

'I'll be here,' I assured everyone, as if they even needed to ask at all.

It would have been both easy and understandable for me to pause the event for the festive period. Pretty much everything else shut down, and as the time trial was free then why shouldn't I? As I explained to anyone who pressed me, it would also have been at odds with my pledge. When I said that I would be there every Saturday, I had meant every word.

Some asked how Jo put up with it, and it was a good question. Right from the start, though, she recognized that this was a commitment I felt I needed to make without compromise. I knew that I could be single-minded. Jo had seen that for herself in my efforts to prepare for the marathon of my life. I also knew how fortunate I was that she could be so understanding. We sometimes joked that as a psychiatric nurse she had another patient in me, but in truth her empathy and patience gave me the space I needed to be myself. While Jo enjoyed the time trial, spending time with friends as a runner and a helper, she also provided me with the space I needed to make it work. This quickly spilled beyond a Saturday morning processing results. After work during the week, I would often return home and rush to my computer to tweak or refine the system. Growth was small but steady, which was fine by me as it allowed me to keep on top of things. At the same time my focus was on making sure that I could continue to cope if the numbers kept tracking upwards. In that period, keen to pitch the time trial as a shared event, I also started a newsletter. I sent it out every Monday, which basically amounted to a run report for the weekend's event. Mindful of my early years as a runner in Johannesburg, where the clubs often relied on print media to publish details of a forthcoming time trial, I included the local newspapers in my dispatch. I even attached photographs from the event each time, aiming to provide everything they needed for a little article. It came to nothing, but that didn't stop me from sending it to the news desk without fail on the first day of every week.

By the time the holiday season arrived, it wasn't just Jo who acknowledged that I could be persistent. On Christmas morning, I hoped that it was seen as a virtue by those runners who trusted me to be waiting in the car park when they could have been at home in festive sweaters and a glass of buck's fizz in hand.

Jo was nervous that nobody would want to do a time trial on Christmas Day. She had started taking part in them with Tim the springer spaniel at her side, and indeed since October the pair had become regulars. Only one of us had picked up an injury after we tripped over each other at the mob match, and it had been great to see my dog continuing to take part in an activity with Jo that we once both loved to do together. It also encouraged others to bring their dogs, which was something I supported wholeheartedly. It tied in with my belief that there should be no obstacles to joining in, and if people would have otherwise stayed at home because they couldn't bring their dog then I would have failed. I even had no issue with dogs running off lead as long as they were as well behaved as their owners. Since starting the time trial, I had come to view it as a playground for runners of every age and ability. If some wanted to race against the clock, as has been my initial assumption, then they had every opportunity to shoot for a personal best. For others, and this had come as a pleasant surprise to me, here was a chance to run for fun in good company that could include their four-legged friends. There was no entry qualification. Age, ability (and breed when it came to the canines) was irrelevant. All that mattered was enthusiasm. For me, that had become the key to making it work. As each Saturday morning event had shown me, there really was room for everyone.

That morning, I had brought Tim with me in a helping capacity. I was grateful to him for the company, thinking this might be the first weekend when people had better things to do.

'Merry Christmas,' I said to my dog, having thrown him the gift of yet another stick.

'And to you, Paul.'

I turned on my heels to find the first arrival in running gear and a Santa hat. Just then, I couldn't have wished for anything more.

By the time I stepped up to give a festive run briefing ahead of the start, twenty-six individuals had grouped together before me to start their Christmas with a time trial. At a time traditionally reserved for families, it felt like I had created one of my own for a lap of the park before everyone returned to their respective homes to make the most of the day. With Jo beside me to help out, cheering the runners as they streamed along the path, it didn't feel like work. I had brought people together. As someone who had known loneliness, that seemed like something to be treasured.

As Christmas Day fell on a Saturday, so too did New Year's Day. Once again, in response to the question and in my newsletter on the morning after Boxing Day, I made it clear that the Bushy Park Time Trial would be taking place as usual.

On this occasion, however, as I announced at the start line a week later having arrived dressed in a tuxedo and trainers, there would be just a slight change to the programme for the first time trial of 2005.

'This morning,' I said, having noted that everyone present was wearing a watch, 'you'll be timing yourselves.'

I paused to let people glance at one another and look perplexed before spelling out why I was dressed for a special event. I was a long way from returning to competitive running, but felt confident that what I had in mind here wouldn't disrupt my recovery.

'I've heard this thing can be fun,' I said, and began to

retreat from them all by several steps. 'So, I thought I'd give it a shot and see what all the fuss is about.'

This time, with no pause to allow them time to register what I had in mind, I counted down from three while spinning around and breaking for the path.

'*Go!*' I yelled gleefully, preparing to be swamped, and didn't stop laughing with the friends who had supported me in getting this community up and running and who I made along the way.

21

FINDING OUR FEET

There is something quietly magical about routine activity. It helps to keep us fit, but also provides structure to our lives. When that activity is enjoyable, and connects us with other people, that can have as much of an impact on our mental wellbeing as it does on our physical health.

As the weeks, months and seasons passed, I found that my Saturday mornings became a high point. At Vodafone, my efforts to make a positive impression had led to me being retained for a bigger and much longer-term project. It meant extended hours from Monday to Friday, and also commuting to and from the company's HQ some fifty miles from home. As a result, weekends were more precious than ever. At nine o'clock sharp, starting the run from the car park, the weight of my working week just fell away.

With experience, I found that overseeing each run became more natural to me. As participants became familiar with how the time trial worked, the more I could relax and enjoy it as a social gathering.

Every time, I saw a few new faces. Some of those would become regulars and in due course I grew to know them all. It felt like a privilege and also a joy to see people forging friendships with each other. Slowly but steadily, the weekly gathering increased in size. By the start of 2006, I could expect to see off over a hundred people from the start line. One year later, that number had almost trebled. In that time, when the uncanny streak of dry Saturday mornings came to an end and we finally ran in the pouring rain, it didn't deter the numbers one little bit.

At my local hardware store, I figured I had become solely responsible for picking clean all the washer stocks from the shelves. As for my number-stamping skills, improving with every session, I could have found work as an engraver.

Throughout, I didn't consider the rising weekly attendance figures as a measure of success. It had a bearing on the system, of course, and led me to keep stamping more washers as if I was coining a new currency. What really made an impression on me was that my event continued to attract runners of all abilities. Most visibly, the time trial had become popular with local running clubs. Every Saturday morning, lean, leggy athletes wearing team vests warmed up before the start. That was fine by me. After all, I had designed the event to be a performance measure for anyone who wished to use it that way. At the same time, people were showing up who looked a little uncertain, or even asked my permission to be there as if somehow there was a qualification for entry. I quickly put them at their ease, and stressed in my briefing that the Bushy Park

Time Trial was open to all. I might have had a narrow view of what defined a runner when I first came up with the idea, but that was broadening by the week and making me very happy. I just hadn't anticipated that running for sheer fun might become the primary driver for so many, and potentially more rewarding. Whatever their reasons for joining me, I just wanted people to have a good time while being active.

'However long it takes you to get round, I'll be here,' I reminded them all. 'It's a run and not a race.'

As the numbers grew from one week to the next, so too did the diversity of participants in terms of age and ability. Some arrived who told me that they hadn't run since their school days. They'd heard about what I was doing and felt comfortable giving it a shot. Knowing as I did that running could transform lives, that was music to my ears. A few brought their parents out of running retirement to join them. Mothers and fathers took turns to lace up their trainers or look after the baby. Others ran while pushing prams or trying to keep up with their young sons or daughters. Then there was the canine contingency, which was always a sight and sound to behold. It was a happy kind of chaos, with a run at the heart of it as an ice breaker for conversation, laughter and forging bonds beyond the finish line. There, seemingly bathed in an endorphin glow from completing five kilometres, people from different pockets of the community made friends.

Over the course of almost three years, I continued to welcome anyone who wanted to join us. I set no rules, and from that grew a mutual respect within the time trial community. There was also no pecking order. The front runners would often finish and then cheer everyone in, while those who clearly found it a challenge received the noisiest reception of all as they approached the finishing funnel. Everyone had their reasons for being there, and benefited from the experience whether they were running or helping me. I never found myself alone on a Saturday morning, and was so grateful to people for their generosity. Talking to Jo, who lent a hand whenever she could, I came to realize that volunteering was perhaps key to the future growth of the time trial. Even though I'd established it as something I could stage without help, that was no longer viable. Those who gave their time to assist me were invaluable, and I wanted to recognize this. As a result, I started to make a note of every person who stepped up, thanked them by name in the newsletter and encouraged anyone to discover that it could be as rewarding as running itself.

In response, I soon came to count on at least a dozen volunteers each weekend. That was enough for me to station people around the course as marshals, and feel confident that I could handle the increasing numbers. It was just a lovely, kind and supportive environment, and I was thrilled to see it thrive.

Before starting the time trial, I had thought long and hard about taking the concept to a running club. It would have been the sensible thing to do in terms of working with an organization with experience in this field. What persuaded me to go it alone came back to my belief that the event should be open to all. Since finding my feet in the UK, in the aftermath of my marriage, I had met some wonderful club runners. Many had become friends, and helped me to pick up the pieces of my life. Essentially I wanted to recreate that environment outside of a club structure so others could benefit who might otherwise miss out. Even if the club had recognized this, and played a low-key role, I still felt that by association it would put off some people from taking part. I hadn't anticipated quite how broad an appeal the time trial would have. It was a pleasant surprise, and only encouraged me to feel like I was taking things in the right direction. While some from the club community had been uncomfortable with my project, fearing it would drain the volunteer pool for their Sunday races or draw runners when they should be resting, they soon came to recognize the time trial was an asset. There was no obligation on anyone to sprint for the finish with their eyeballs on stalks, and indeed many runners with a fixture the next day treated it as an enjoyable shake down with friends. As for the volunteers, the clubs saw their numbers increase as those who helped out at the time trials came to realize that being involved in any kind of running event brought its own rewards.

I would like to say that everyone was happy. In reality, there came a point where I couldn't ignore some voices of concern. While people were supportive of my weekly gathering in the park, it was becoming increasingly evident as it grew that I was at risk of tripping over red tape.

'Paul, have you thought about insurance?'

The question seemed to crop up with increasing frequency. Mostly it was asked by people from a running club background. As a formality, any club event would require some kind of coverage against legal liabilities such as injury or property damage. There was no way they could let even one runner loose without it, and here I was with several hundred on my watch.

'Yes,' I said each time, though anyone just had to look into my eyes to know that behind my literal answer I'd gone no further than contemplating it.

As I saw things, insurance was just another potential obstacle I had tried to avoid. My main concern was that an insurer might dictate how I was running the time trial, when I had gone to great lengths to keep things simple. My view was that everyone should be responsible for themselves, and that it would be unthinkable for anybody to seek financial compensation from what was essentially a free run in the park. There was no commercial motivation here. Nobody was making any money from the venture. At the same time, as people pointed out, there was still a risk at large in not covering myself for all eventualities. As much as I saw the time trial as a bubble of goodness that brought out the best in everyone, I had to be realistic. Should the worst occur, it wasn't an argument that would work in my defence before a judge.

So, with great reluctance and having held out for as long as I could, I agreed to place the time trial on a formal footing. I intended to cover the cost of the policy myself when I found one that worked for me, as I had for the various bits and pieces that allowed me to run the event. It was a small price to pay for the happiness that the time trial seemed to create, for me as much as everyone who got involved. Apart from the washers, I had invested in a few cones as we had started marking out the whole course. With so many runners, it had felt like the right thing to do. I also acquired a roll of tape and stakes to create a finishing funnel that could cope with the larger numbers, but perhaps my biggest outlay was for a laptop. It might have been an increasingly commonplace piece of tech at the time, but it wasn't cheap. Still, as it meant I could process the results from the cafe after each time trial, I saw it as money well spent. It meant I could stay for longer at what I came to consider as the true finish line: namely the upper floor of the Caffè Nero in Teddington that we informally took over for an hour or so every Saturday morning.

As for my well-meaning friends, they were both pleased and relieved when I begrudgingly agreed to look into an insurance policy, and yet they still had questions.

'You have permission to use the park, right?' they asked, as if perhaps that should have been the first thing to secure.

Naturally I assured them it was all in hand.

It wasn't.

My assumption had been that a royal park meant it was open to the people. It was probably fine when I started, as an informal gathering of a few friends and fellow runners for a lap around the park. In my bid to stay under the radar, we were gone by ten o'clock. We left no trace of our presence, and only afterwards did the paths and car parks really start to fill. However, the weekly time trial had now grown to a size that was hard to ignore. During spring and autumn, when the ground was wet underfoot, the short grass stretches on the course quickly degraded to mud under the feet of hundreds of runners. In particular, this applied to the stretch in the funnel I had created with the tape and stakes to ensure people crossed the line one at a time for position purposes. Then there was the local paper. Having ignored my weekly run report for years, at last it had started to feature in print. I'd been submitting one after every event, seemingly into the abyss. When it first appeared I read it as a validation not just of the time trial but my persistence. We were no longer under the radar, and so I decided that the time had come to reach out to the park officials in case they reached out to me first with a view to kicking us off.

Shortly after my friends had broached the subject, I arranged a meeting with the park ranger. He worked from a beautiful lodge house in Bushy Park, and an audience with him had required an appointment. As the ranger's office operated on business hours only, I'd had to take time off work at Vodafone and drive home early for a late afternoon meeting. It all contributed to my feeling that it was just a hassle I had been right to avoid, coupled with a slight sense of intimidation when the receptionist at the lodge house invited me to take a seat.

Ten minutes after our appointed meeting time, sensing I'd been made to wait deliberately and sweat it out, the ranger appeared at his office door.

'Mr Sinton-Hewitt?' he said, in a way that left me in no doubt that he knew full well it was me. 'Pleased to meet you at last.'

In full uniform, the ranger was a giant of a man. He was well over six foot, but may have seemed tall to me because just then I felt uncomfortably small. This guy was in charge of a prestigious park, and for several years now I had been spinning runners around it every Saturday morning like I owned it all. Even before he settled behind his desk and invited me to take a chair in front of it, I was embarrassed at my lack of etiquette. I should have asked permission, and now here I was hoping to secure it long after the fact.

'So, you may have heard of my time trial,' I began. 'It starts and finishes in the car park near the fountain.'

The guy regarded me impassively, as if waiting for me to keep digging until I hit the rock bed. Holding his gaze across the desk, I explained that it wasn't a commercial venture. No money changed hands. We didn't put up signs or leave a mess. We were respectful of other park users, such as cyclists and horse riders, and indeed the only thing I felt I needed to apologize for was that it had taken me so long to introduce myself.

'So, that's why I'm here,' I said to finish, and then heard myself continue to speak as if my mouth had just secured independence from my brain. 'In case you weren't aware of it.'

This time, the ranger responded with a flicker of amusement in his expression. He sat back in his chair, still considering me.

'You really think I don't know what you've been doing?' he asked.

I looked to my shoes, mindful that the sight of a small army of runners tooling around the pathways at the same time every week must be quite hard to miss.

'I suppose you might have had an idea,' I confessed, before facing him once again. 'Maybe you should join us? Everyone who comes has a great time!'

Seemingly deaf to my invitation, the ranger opened the desk drawer in front of him. In that moment, judging by the small smile he tried keep to himself, I knew that he always had every intention of granting permission. He'd just been making me pay for the fact that I hadn't involved him from the start. Even then, I knew that had I approached him with a proposal, it wouldn't have come close to illustrating the sheer joy to be had every Saturday morning that he had no doubt seen for himself. If anything, I thought to myself, he would have sent me away. Instead, I watched him produce a form from the drawer.

'If you want to continue then you have to fill in an application,' he said, and pushed it across the desk. 'It's the same rule for everyone. You're not a special case, Mr Sinton-Hewitt!'

'Understood,' I said, feeling suddenly relieved. 'Is that it?'

'That's it,' he said, rising to his feet as if to signal the meeting was now closed.

I stood up, collecting the form.

'Thank you,' I said. 'I'm so glad we've finally met.'

In response, as if something outstanding had just sounded an alarm in his mind, the ranger's eyes narrowed by a jot.

'You do have insurance?' he asked.

'From the moment I started,' I assured him, upon which it jumped to the top of my to-do list before we'd even shaken hands.

22

A DOG WITH A BONE

When I began the Bushy Park Time Trial, there was no doubt in my mind that it would run and run. Even if nobody showed up, I would never walk away. That was the basis for the event. I set out to create something people could rely on and which they could use as they saw fit. It was a church, of sorts. That door would always be open.

Initially, I thought runners might take part occasionally, and over time that would create a steady number from one weekend to the next. As it became evident that the numbers gathering in the car park were gradually creeping up, I tried to stay one step ahead. Despite my best efforts to keep stamping enough washers, I could still run short whenever the steady rise in popularity spiked. That prompted a hurried back-up system that involved handing finishers scraps of paper with their finishing position, but we managed all the same.

Despite my efforts to make sure the system could cater for all eventualities, when it began to creak I knew we had to take things to the next level. My application to the park authorities had secured permission for us to be there, and I'd turned to England Athletics for insurance cover. As the governing body for athletics in the country, I was well aware that my time trial was unconventional. There was no membership requirement or coaching opportunities for aspiring or talented athletes like there was at the clubs and organizations they traditionally recognized. Nor was it a race. My event was just an opportunity for everyday people to be active on a regular basis. I was also just some upstart who happened to be persistent, appealing to their obligation to support community engagement. At first, it was suggested that insurance could only be issued if each time trial was attended by St John's Ambulance. That just wasn't going to happen. For one thing, I had no money to fund that kind of service on a weekly basis. I just had a growing and enthusiastic community who enjoyed running together on a Saturday morning.

To be fair to England Athletics, they agreed to issue the policy I needed once I'd undertaken a health and safety review. I had already asked that dogs should run on leads – which deep down I knew to be inevitable but had been fun while it lasted – while the review led to the introduction of a minimum age of four for children. The latter went against the grain of my belief that on principle the time trial should be open to absolutely everybody. It was also a compromise I realized I would have to make, which marked a rising sense that I was beginning to face complexities in sustaining the event. Sweatshop were still generously providing me with weekly prizes in the form of vouchers for the first and last runner, and would continue to do so for quite some time. The time trial was driving sales at their local store, but it was another working relationship that I found myself depending on to help the venture thrive.

As the event continued to grow in popularity, so too did the demand on my time. Throughout, my responsibilities to the project at Vodafone were mounting. I was managing a team of people, and working to tight schedules. It left me exhausted at the end of each day, and yet I'd return home to a list of things I needed to do to keep the time trial running. In my constant bid to make it as accessible as possible, I cobbled together a website. It was basic but functional. At *bptt.net*, people could view their results for the week and even access the archive. My aim was to provide people with as much data as possible in a way that could be easily understood.

The website hadn't taken me long to create, and frankly it showed. What kept me up until the early hours was coding and managing the results database. I was still updating and then printing a list of everyone who had ever taken part in a time trial. By the summer of 2006, I was greeting 200 to 300 participants each week from a database containing over 2,000 entries. Before the start, when I asked for first-timers to make their presence known, a sizeable show of hands would tell me that the blank pages at the back of the list in the boot of my car would be completely filled. Later, in front of my laptop in the cafe, and afterwards in my office at home, I would have to manually input all the new names and contact details into the database. It was fiddly and intensive work, on top of having to email the results, but also the only way that I could keep simplicity at the heart of what I was offering. I could have switched to a pre-registration system, but at that moment in time it seemed off-putting. Participants just had to show up and run. I didn't want to place anything in their way that might deter them, even if that meant sacrificing time I would otherwise spend with Jo and the family.

'I'm a time trial widow,' she would say from time to time, and though she did so with a smile I felt bad.

The fact was she had a point. I had started something that was now taking me away from someone really important to me. Since we'd got together, I felt grounded, happy and loved. I strived to offer Jo the same thing, but what I couldn't provide was time. Fortunately, and to my endless gratitude, she recognized this was something I needed to do, and which even brought out the best in me. Ultimately, it was no reflection of my commitment to her, but something I could only do because of her generosity of spirit. It helped that Jo was closely involved in the time trial. She ran and volunteered whenever she could, often joined by her young son and daughter, and became a valuable confidante in helping me to develop ideas. Jo and I became a team. Without her, I couldn't have provided the commitment to a weekly event that it needed in order to flourish.

What I never anticipated, however, was that I could replicate the time trial in other parks. With my consultancy work to consider, I was running on fumes. I had set out to create a single event in Bushy Park. Three years on, its popularity had taken me completely by surprise. I loved the experience, but when the suggestion was made that I could start a second time trial I had only one response.

'It's out of the question,' I insisted. 'There's only one of me.'

As the event had taken off at Bushy Park, I'd often been asked if I would put on a 10K version. I had ruled that out from the start for several reasons. Firstly, it would only take away resources from what I had up and running. More immediately, I knew that would present competition to the clubs and commercial companies who staged races of that distance. I didn't want to step on their toes, especially as I'd worked so hard to bring the clubs round to the belief that the time trial presented no threat. At the same time, I firmly believed that nobody should pay to run a 5K just for fun. It just struck me as money for nothing, and I was quite happy to curtail that with my free, weekly event. Ultimately, my focus was on making sure that Bushy Park remained robust in the face of rising numbers. If I set up a second time trial, the expenses would only increase when I already felt like I was in the red at home in terms of time.

It was my friend, Jim Desmond, who first raised the question with me. Since the start of the time trial at Bushy Park, he acknowledged that I had started something with the potential to make a difference. He ran and volunteered on a regular basis, and I also came to consider him as one of my unofficial consultants. Together with Jo, Duncan Gaskell and whoever happened to be around the table in the pub, we would pick apart what was working with the time trial and the things that needed attention. The great thing about a weekly event, as I quickly came to realize, was that we could quickly implement refinements and changes. An annual marathon would have to wait a year to improve things. We could have it implemented within seven days. This way, following a headache with the results processing one Saturday, we had quickly introduced a way to ensure that the timing and position data matched up by stationing a volunteer at the funnel exit with a pen and paper. By jotting down names and washer number at regular intervals, our 'number checker' could provide us with a means to isolate any discrepancy in the results and swiftly resolve it. We even redesigned the course to accommodate the bigger numbers, all of which could be done where necessary in the space of seven days. Jim was always making suggestions to fine-tune the process, just like everyone else, but when it came to replicating the event in another park he was like a dog with a bone.

'You can do more, Paul. The demand is there.'

I had no doubt that people would respond to another time trial as they had at Bushy Park. But as I reminded him, repeatedly, I couldn't be in two places at once.

'If somebody else wants to set one up then be my guest,' I said. 'It's just a group run on a Saturday morning. Anybody can start one from scratch.'

'There's more to it than that,' Jim insisted, and I knew he was talking about the community that had sprung up around it. The time trial had evolved to become about family, whatever that meant to different people, from the runners to the volunteers. Something unexpected and unique had emerged from the event, like a chemical reaction I hadn't foreseen, and it brought everyone together. That was special to me, but I was well aware that it meant just as much to others for all sorts of reasons. We had something precious, and I worried about just what it would take to replicate. In turning my attention to a second event, and finding I'd spread myself too thinly, I could potentially let everyone down. Jim Desmond heard me out. But he refused to let it go. Instead, he set about revising his pitch to me in a way that rendered all my concerns redundant.

In the autumn of 2006, as I sat down with a pint and my casual advisory board to celebrate what would be the third year since starting the Bushy Park Time Trial, Jim presented me with a forward plan in the form of a map that he had sketched.

'This is the course for Wimbledon Common,' said Jim, referring to another green space just up the road from where we lived. 'I've been out and measured it properly with the trundle wheel. It's exactly 5K, with plenty of space to start and finish, and a cafe that serves coffee and cake. Everyone here thinks it's a great idea, and you'll get all the support you need from us to make it work.' Jim stopped there and tapped on the table with one finger as if to be sure he had my full attention. 'All you have to do is say yes.'

I stared at the map in front of me for a moment longer. Then I looked up. Around the table, people were waiting for me to say something. I stood by the fact that I couldn't start another event on my own. It would be too much. If it was going to work, it would require commitment not just from my friends but also the wider community. In this light, having seen how Bushy Park had brought out the best in people, from the enthusiasm for a shared passion to the mutual support, camaraderie and encouragement among runners and volunteers every weekend, all I could do was settle my gaze on the man who had just got me over the line and then smile.

'A toast,' I said, raising my glass and waiting for everyone else to follow suit. 'To Wimbledon Common Time Trial.'

23

IT'LL ALL COME GOOD IN THE END

Trust has always been important to me. It stemmed from a time in my life when that was lacking. When it came to launching the second time trial, I knew that I could rely on Jim. He understood what I had set out to achieve, and helped me to make sure the moving parts supported it. Six weeks after I agreed to give it a shot, we had assembled a team of local time trial enthusiasts to help bring the magic of a free, weekly timed run to Wimbledon Common.

This time, I did everything by the book. We sought permission from the park authorities and extended the insurance cover. Rather than slip under the red tape, we established a process that worked through every step to place the second time trial on solid foundations. In front of my computer, I opened up the system I'd created and adapted it to cater for two time trials. Both events would share the same database, I decided, as I thought it would be great if registered participants could just show up and run at either one. I was well aware that it meant the database would just grow even bigger, and potentially unwieldy for me to manage, but it seemed like one more step towards making it as simple as possible for people to get involved.

I was present for the first two weekends at Wimbledon, in a supporting role to Jim and his volunteers while Duncan Gaskell and a small band of friends took up the reins at Bushy Park. I had every confidence that Jim could deliver the event. While the first one had taken over my life very quickly, Jo and I had still entrusted it into his care for a couple of weekends when we took a much-needed holiday. We had travelled all the way to New Zealand, in fact, as a fiftieth birthday surprise for my old running friend, Noel DeCharmoy who had emigrated there from South Africa. Jim had proven to be a natural run director in my absence, with Duncan working alongside him to create a dependable double act. It proved to me that others could fulfil my role and even do a better job. Ultimately, this led me to believe that the Wimbledon Common time trial could work. When it came to the launch, we kept it purposely low-key to be sure that we could cope. Fifty-one runners showed up for the first event. The following Saturday, that number grew to fifty-six and the volunteers doubled to four. It was exactly the kind of turnout we'd been hoping for, with signs of a quiet momentum, and I left Jim and the team knowing that the event was in good hands.

Back at Bushy Park, where close to 400 runners filed through the finishing funnel every week, I began to look at the event in a different light. Wimbledon seemed set to prove to me that the time trial could be replicated without compromise. The communal spirit couldn't be manufactured. We just set the framework that allowed it to grow, and then celebrated the fact that it brought out the best in everybody. The black fleece jacket I had taken to wearing with pride for each event was a case in point. It had been presented to me by a group of kind-hearted runners to mark the one-hundredth time trial. As a complete surprise to me, they had customized the top so it was emblazoned on the breast pocket with BPTT and my name across the shoulders. I thought it was terrific. I took great pride in wearing it every week, and it made me think I could do something similar for people when they hit the same milestone.

Soon after the jacket was presented to me, a handful of regulars who had been with me since the early days were close to completing one hundred time trials at the park. It was one thing for me to turn up and then stand around with a stopwatch at each event, but quite another to run so many of them. With that it mind, I ordered ten jackets like mine, but with '100' printed across the back. Darren Wood was the first to receive the milestone jacket, with several more coming out of the box in quick succession. It was such a joy to mark the achievement. I was just conscious that it was also another outlay from my pocket in expenses that were beginning to mount. Realistically, I would struggle to keep covering the cost if people reached the same milestone, but it wasn't the only reason why I realized that financing the venture could become an issue.

In order to set up the second time trial, I'd had to buy resources for course-marking and a laptop for the team to process results. Sometime earlier, concerned that I was exceeding the goodwill extended by Ranelagh Harriers in letting me borrow their stopwatch, I had invested in one of my own. Now I found myself buying another one, and wondering where it would end. For just as the financial outlay began to reach a point where I was reluctant to put a precise figure on it for Jo, so I couldn't shake the idea that perhaps we had a format for an event that could take off elsewhere. I began to see it as an investment not in financial terms but happiness. Bushy Park Time Trial had saved me during a challenging period, and I saw what a difference it made to others in all sorts of ways. I couldn't put a price on it. Just as the internet had evolved to a point where we could make new and exciting connections in a virtual world, this was a means to bring people together in a way that we seemed to have lost. It encouraged them to get up, get out and enjoy a shared activity. That was good for hearts and minds, I realized, while the steady rise in enthusiasm for what I had started told me that eventually it would draw attention from the private or public sector with the means to fund it. With this in mind, I decided that it had to be worth putting my hand in my pocket for a further roll-out to showcase what a good thing we had going.

By now, three years into the venture, the time trial had overtaken my life. It had also given rise to a heartfelt belief that it was a force for good. I might have founded it for selfish reasons, as an injured runner seeking company, but had then quickly discovered the rewards to be had from encouraging others to bring out the best in themselves. In response, those that had gathered at the start line for all sorts of reasons showed me the potential was limitless. It wasn't just about chasing personal bests, I now recognized with absolute conviction, but getting people outdoors, active and social.

Over time, this whole project had become a mission that I'd never foreseen. With no long-term planning in place when I had started, it created demands on me that I struggled to meet. To establish new events, I would need to rely on inviting people on board who recognized that investing time in making it work brought rewards for their communities. Mulling things over in my mind, I began to hatch a plan. I knew that I could provide the knowledge, training and expertise for anyone who wanted a time trial in their area. In return, I would encourage those organizers to assemble their own teams, raise a small fund from local sponsors, grants or donations to cover the cost of essential items like a laptop, stopwatch, cones, tokens and tape, and then effectively run the event themselves. As well as bringing them up to speed, I would be on call to provide help and advice. I would also continue to look after the system that handled the database and processed results, as well as the website that published them every week. When I next sat down in the pub with my friends and shared the plan, everyone recognized that both the demand and support existed for this cookie-cutter model. What they questioned, as I had anticipated, was how I planned to pay for it. While event teams recognized the need to raise start-up funds, which gave communities a stake in the event, I still faced considerable operating costs. Frankly, I wasn't sure how deep my pockets could be. There were limits after all. I just had to place my faith in the fact that doing something with goodness at its heart would ultimately draw support.

'It'll all work out in the end,' I said. 'We just have to keep doing the right thing.'

From that moment on, events progressed rapidly. It was as if momentum had built to a point where the advances became exponential. While I returned to my keyboard to customize the front and back-end system I'd originally built to support one time trial and soup it up for more, my friends began to mobilize their running contacts in a bid to spread the word. We had proven that the format worked. Now we needed teams to establish time trials in new parks and open spaces. Most who stepped up had taken part in a time trial at Bushy Park or Wimbledon Common. They understood what it could offer, and if anyone was interested who hadn't run one then we invited them to come along and experience it for themselves. In my view, the most effective way to pitch the concept to people was by asking them to join in. That didn't just apply to those who would go on to start new time trials. Now there was some urgency to funding the whole venture, I approached potential backers by inviting them to throw on their running gear for a community run that could take us all places.

As a strategy it worked.

By the end of 2007, seven time trials had sprung into existence. First Banstead Woods in Surrey joined Bushy Park and Wimbledon Common, followed by Hyde Park, Richmond Park, Bramhall Park, Cardiff Park, Albert Park and Brighton and Hove. Altogether, over 800 people were taking part on a weekly basis. A year later, that number had climbed to 1,500 across fifteen time trials including events in Scotland and Wales. Thankfully, I also managed to secure a small amount of funding so that I could at least sleep at night. It felt like quite a step up, but a necessary one as everything was growing at such a fast rate. Inevitably, bringing in what I had to accept was sponsorship presented issues that needed some negotiation. I sought companies that felt like a good fit with the spirit of the time trials, and recognized what so many people saw in them. Right from the start, however, I was quite clear that the events could not be bought or hijacked to sell products. It was about promoting health and wellbeing, with any benefit to those backers coming from being associated with a good thing. I was well aware that my position was entrenched, and inevitably that meant those early relationships did not last as long as they might otherwise have done. The money was important, but so too were the values that brought everyone together every Saturday morning. It was a community, not a commercial prospect, and as yet more time trials came into existence I held out in the belief that it could be funded without compromise.

As well as building links with sponsors, I set about applying for all manner of different grants. It was intensive work, and I just had to carve out time to get it done. I was also aware that I needed to look professional. That meant pulling data into presentations so I could demonstrate with figures what a good thing we had going. After much discussion at the pub, and the realization that I needed to account for the funding trickling in, I created a limited company and determined that it should be run as a not-for-profit. If we ever reached a point where income exceeded costs, it would just be reinvested into the venture.

'It's called UK Time Trials Ltd,' I reported back, having registered the name.

My aim had been to capture all the time trials under one banner. With more people coming forward to start another handful of events across the country, it seemed appropriate to me. And also rather neat. Around the table, however, my friends seemed underwhelmed. Some even questioned if the term 'time trial' reflected the true nature of the event as it had evolved, though everyone was keen to see how things would develop.

Around the same time, I made a decision that was both scary and exciting. It had become increasingly clear to me that the decision to expand created more work than I could manage. Each event required me to stamp 200 washers, along with the constant need to keep supplying replacements. It was also just the start of my responsibilities. Every Friday, having made sure the database of all the participants was up to date, I'd email copies to each event team leader for them to print out and take along to the time trial in the morning. Later that day, when they returned the timing and position files I needed along with a whole sheaf of first-timer details, it would all need inputting into the system before I could process and release the results for each event. Increasingly, it all became quite an undertaking involving caffeine, reams of printouts and patience.

Week in, week out, it was fiddly, time-consuming work that was also prone to error. Ultimately, I knew that I needed to find the time to create a better system. With my commitment to Vodafone, however, there simply weren't enough hours in the day. I couldn't afford to quit in order to fully commit to UK Time Trials, but what I could do,

I realized, was take a chunk from my salary as well as some of the sponsorship money and employ someone to help me. It was a big financial commitment, which meant I had to be entirely transparent with Jo. On a practical level, it meant we would have to tighten our belts at home. I saw no other way to act on my conviction that we were growing something very special here. I also knew that if I didn't pursue this course then the system would become overwhelmed with the growing numbers. It could even threaten the existence of the time trials. As someone who had been at my side since I first came up with the idea, and enjoyed running at the events and volunteered regularly, Jo saw it was a sacrifice worth making.

Somehow, I promised her, it would be an investment.

When it came to who to bring on board, I had just one person in mind. Chris Wright was a regular volunteer at Bushy Park Time Trial. Known to one and all as 'Crispy' – as his middle name began with the letter P and nobody could ignore how that sounded – he had always struck me as being meticulous when it came to detail. In setting up the course, everything had to be just right through his eyes, which was in contrast to my tendency to focus on the bigger picture. We made a good pair, and so when I learned that he had just come onto the job market I invited him on board.

'Come and work for me,' I said. 'Join the UK Time Trial team.'

Crispy went away to give it some thought, and I didn't blame him given that my pitch to him was fuelled by a dream rather than a solid business plan. Still, I was delighted when he accepted the opportunity. As soon as he got involved, I knew I had made the right decision. Crispy was brilliant at diligently assembling all the paperwork and documentation that had previously taken up so much of my time. It freed me up to forge contacts with potential sponsors, bring new event teams up to speed and ultimately spend time reinventing a results system that I had only ever intended to use to manage a single weekly event.

In doing so, I made what should have felt like a concession but instead proved to be a liberation.

I had wanted to remain with the registration model that encouraged people to take part in an event and write down their details afterwards, but frankly it was becoming untenable. The rise in new sign-ups was too great, and also unpredictable in volume from one week to the next. As the internet continued to establish a place in our world, I recognized that registering online in advance could in fact be more attractive to participants than queuing up after finishing to scribble on a clipboard.

From the week I introduced the change, giving first-timers until 6 p.m. on a Friday to register for an event the next morning, life at the back end of the system became more bearable. With Crispy shouldering the load in other areas, at last it felt like I was catching up with something that had been in danger of running away from me. We each played to our own strengths, and Crispy's contribution could not be underestimated. Even if I didn't always recognize it at the time.

'Have you ever considered changing the name?' he asked me, early on in our partnership, and voiced the same concerns about the Time Trial monicker as so many of my friends. It wasn't ideal, given how the events encouraged people to get involved for all sorts of reasons, but then nor did it strike me as something that held us back in any way. Only recently had another volunteer – a lovely, insightful and disarmingly frank guy called Stuart Lodge – added his name to the list of people who questioned if the 'time trial' concept truly captured the communal spirit of what the event had become. Unlike everyone else, however, he had also come up with a suggestion of his own. Having bluntly told me that in his view the current name was 'shit', Stuart had proposed something like *Park Run* might be more appealing to the broad range of people it was drawing in every Saturday morning.

'Why would I change something that's not broken,' I said to Crispy, as I had to Stuart, and quietly hoped he would just focus his attention on the work stuff where he really shone. We were shooting for the moon here, after all. The rocket had successfully lifted from the launch pad, and we were on our way. It seemed to me a little late and unnecessary to be fretting over the name of the mission.

Without my sole employee, working so diligently on articles of association or writing up processes for new teams to follow, I would not have been able to focus my efforts on securing backing that had to support our aims. In 2008, in a moment that I could barely believe was happening, I signed a partnership deal with Nike. They really seemed to understand why people were drawn to the venture, and committed to helping me develop it. As well as a welcome financial contribution, which meant I didn't need to keep funding new time trials from my own pocket, the company generously hooked me up with their marketing team.

Straight away, they understood our values, aims and ambitions. They were smart, young and hip, and wholeheartedly embraced the idea that milestones should be celebrated. They proposed switching from a black fleece to a snappier, more economically viable t-shirt in the same colour, and expanding the milestone range so we didn't just celebrate one hundred runs. In addition, we'd offer a white t-shirt to children who completed ten time trials, and a red one for anyone who reached fifty. I loved the fact that it made milestones achievable for everyone, even if it was still no mean feat for so many. There was just one sticking point, as I learned at the meeting where the marketing team had presented me with their designs.

'It's the name,' said the guy leading the pitch, who suddenly seemed a little sheepish. 'Time Trial is a bit, well . . .'

'Shit?' I suggested, echoing Stuart's opinion and voicing what was clearly on the tip of the guy's tongue.

In response, the entire marketing team looked relieved that I appeared to share their view. Quietly thankful that I hadn't brought Crispy with me to point out that I had just conceded something people had been trying to tell me for ages, I figured I could at least make a constructive suggestion.

'It isn't mine,' I admitted, 'but I think we can work with it.'

The team leader glanced around at his colleagues, as if perhaps to signal that he had to humour me.

'Go on.'

'*Park Run*,' I said, to which everyone seemed to sit up in their seats.

The guy didn't blink for a moment. Then he nodded to himself, and again with more certainty.

'Let's make it a single word,' he proposed, living up to Nike's reputation for design elegance, and promptly raised his hands as if to contain the name he proposed. '*Parkrun*.'

Amid the murmurs of approval, I had just one thing to say.

'Could we drop the capital letter?' I asked, pitching for a more friendly, informal and relaxed expression of the name. I'd also just got my first iPhone, and thought it was a cool thing to do. Even if it would cause me endless grief in years to come, as autocorrect technology stubbornly insisted on capitalizing the name, it seemed like a good idea. Just then, one of the marketeers wrote it out across a whiteboard so we could see how it looked for ourselves.

parkrun

In that moment, as I said it to myself like everyone else around the table, I knew we had a name that needed no explanation. Spelling out something unique and local to everyone, *parkrun* would come to represent the moment a small grass roots community venture tilted towards a social movement.

24

LEAP OF FAITH

After injury ended my marathon dreams, two years passed before I began to ease back into running on a regular basis. This time I had no need for training plans. With so much else going on in my life since I'd been forced to give up on an activity I loved, a sea change had occurred in what it meant to me. I was no longer driven to chase fast times. I still really admired people who pushed themselves as I had, but now I saw things in a different light. Thanks to the communities taking shape in parks around the country on a Saturday morning, I had come to appreciate that running could mean so much more to us all. It didn't just apply to professional athletes and club runners but anyone who recognized that a shared activity such as *parkrun* could bring lasting benefits to our physical and mental welfare. It brought people together, just for a short time every Saturday morning, but that was enough to create a sense of joy, positivity and belonging: something a lost little boy in a children's home had once yearned to experience for himself.

By 2009, five years since I'd first leafleted flyers for a new event in Bushy Park, the journey it had started continued to take us to new places. That October, we'd established a total of almost thirty events around the UK, with an average of 2,500 runners getting involved each weekend and more than 25,000 participants registered on my database. I was still turning around the results from each *parkrun* once they'd returned the data I needed. The switch to online registration made it all so much easier to manage, but the growing number of events still made it time-intensive. Along with all the calls and meetings I had to keep making in my hunt for sponsorship and grants, and even with Crispy taking the strain elsewhere, I knew that I couldn't manage without another member of staff. I was still squeezing in the hours around my consultancy job, but I couldn't afford to pack it in. That was my sole source of income. It paid well, but I wasn't saving anything. After the mortgage and domestic bills, anything left over went into the company. The Nike sponsorship had taken away some of that financial pressure, but *parkrun* wasn't a money-making venture. Nor was I ever tempted to transform it into one. Right from the start, it was very clear to me that we could only grow through the social contract we forged with local communities. This wasn't about getting rich. It was about enriching the lives of people who got involved with *parkrun*, whether as participants or volunteers.

It was one thing to stand my ground and not sell out, but I still had to find a way to place *parkrun* on sound financial footing. One time I totted up all the money I had put into it. The total reached £50,000, which rather took my breath away. All I could do was treat it like an incredibly expensive hobby that made me happy while striving to build financial backing that maintained our values. Much of it came down to faith, and that came from what I saw in each and every event on a weekly basis.

It wasn't easy, but the ever-rising groundswell of goodwill from all the volunteer teams made the effort worthwhile. Crispy and I were as committed as the people who had stepped up to help us grow *parkrun*, and I owed it to them to strengthen the support they received. So, while ignoring my personal bank statements, it was a delight and something of a relief to bring a new member of the team on board. Anita Afonso came highly recommended by our friends at Nike, where she had previously worked in a public-facing role. We needed help in managing and coordinating the rising number of new events, as well as providing an extra pair of hands on deck as we sailed into uncharted waters. Having met Anita to discuss the role, and seen for myself that she was a smart and proactive team player, I knew she would prove invaluable.

Just ahead of her arrival, with so much going on, it became clear to me that I was running a small company that required a headquarters. Mostly, I worked from a cubbyhole under the stairs at home. As Jo and I had four children between us, either teenagers or on the cusp of adulthood, we had quite a revolving door in terms of who stayed with us. Crispy worked from his place nearby, but we also met at mine on a regular basis. In a busy environment, with people coming and going, it wasn't ideal for us to be on phones and laptops at the kitchen table or in the front room. Nor was it viable with a third person set to join the team. On limited time before Anita started, I knew I had to do something.

Sometimes, on the drive home from my consultancy work, which had taken me from Vodafone to Hutchison 3G – another telecommunications giant who were in the process of launching the Three network – I would fantasize about renting the kind of state-of-the-art building I occupied in my day job. It would be lovely, I thought to myself, to operate from a gleaming space constructed from chrome and glass. While that was out of the question, I believed that it would benefit Crispy, Anita and me if we had a workspace we could call our own.

Which is how I turned my attention to the shed in my back garden.

I had constructed it myself several years earlier. Having gained some confidence in converting the loft into a bedroom to create some more space under the roof, I had set my sights on a kind of adult den. It would be more than just a store for tools and the lawn mower, and I had drawn up a plan to build a timber structure that also served as a kind of summer house. When bedlam ruled in the house, it would be a place I could escape to with a coffee and the Sunday papers. That had been the plan. With a very small budget and grand designs, I prepared the foundations and then talked myself into taking delivery of five old telegraph poles. A friend with far better carpentry skills than I possessed helped me in sawing them into the raw materials needed to build the structure. We installed a roof, with windows at each end, but left the dwelling space open in a way that reminded me of the old rondavel of my early years in Johannesburg.

The shed was in no way fit for purpose as a professional working environment, and yet I felt it had potential. Over a couple of weekends, my handyman friend closed up the open plan element and installed both insulation and power. Fortunately, we had been quite generous with the size of the structure. It was way too big for a tool store and a couple of garden chairs, but fitted the bill just fine for my workforce at the time. It even had room, I estimated, to squeeze in one or two more staff should we need it.

That same year, as *parkrun* approached a tipping point, that little space swiftly began to fill. From the shed in my back garden, it felt like we were marshalling a running revolution by the people.

Every year, a popular magazine called *Runner's World* issued a series of awards to individuals for outstanding achievement in the running community. In 2009, out of nowhere, it seemed to us at the time, the magazine included me among the six winners. The supporting article praised *parkrun* as 'the perfect example of grassroots sports participation'. It was a great honour to find myself listed alongside the likes of fell running legend, Joss Naylor and the Olympian Dame Kelly Holmes. In the month that issue of the magazine was published, it also sparked a surge in the number of people who turned up at the events we had recently started around the country. It was an exciting time, but also nerve-wracking. We had avoided taking out any advertising for *parkrun* for two simple reasons. Firstly, we couldn't afford it. More importantly, word of mouth was strong. It generated enough interest to keep the numbers rising at a rate we could manage. We aimed to set up each event to be flexible, but this was uncharted territory. I was anxious that a sudden influx would put an undue strain not just on my results system but also on the teams. It could even leave them unable to cope.

In the wake of the award, the steady rise in *parkrun* participants each week shifted up a gear. Within the space of a year, we were welcoming close to 6,000 runners at almost thirty events. In that time, my concerns about whether it might overload the system proved unfounded both at the back end in the shed and the front end at events around the UK. The volunteer teams stepped up to demonstrate that *parkrun* could welcome one and all. The nearby coffee shops were also delighted by the uptick in custom afterwards. When a new cafe opened within the park at Bushy, a good-natured takeover would take place after each event. By 2010, when I could send off up to 600 people from the start line, the staff would be on battle footing for the influx that followed. My software system also coped with the increase in results for me to turn around, even if I knew that a time would soon come when there wouldn't be enough hours in my day to process everything.

Naturally, people began to ask me if there was a limit to what we could manage. Even then, as new events went live on a regular basis, my view was that we had only just begun. Yes, I was driven by the spirit of idealism, but I genuinely believed that by taking one step at a time and sticking to our core values of community, accessibility and simplicity then our efforts would prove worthwhile. Our family of sponsors was growing and providing the financial stability we needed. It was just a question of ensuring that it could support the rate of growth. So, in the face of the question that would be levelled at me as new events continued to seed and flourish, I had just one answer:

'I want to see a *parkrun* in every community. Every town and village should have one.'

I knew that I was dreaming big. I was also well aware that it was time for me to make one of those life decisions from the heart. If I wanted my ambitions for *parkrun* to become a reality, I would have to commit to it wholeheartedly, and that meant making it my sole occupation. After a career in system software architecture spanning more than twenty years, having reached a place that I loved, I began to think what life would look like if I gave up the consultancy. Having joined Hutchison at a time when *parkrun* was taking off, they had been nothing but supportive. They recognized that it was chewing up my time, and while I had a responsibility to make my work with them a priority I was always having to slip away to make calls or attend meetings. Over the preceding months, as *parkrun* became more pressing, I had dropped from full time to three days a week. It put a squeeze on the projects I had to deliver for them, and also meant I was invoicing them for fewer hours. In some ways, that meant it was easier for me to contemplate the leap of faith I needed to make. I just couldn't quite bring myself to cut all ties from that financial lifeline. Having struggled with my career before striking out on my own as a consultant, did I really want to give it up completely?

It was Jo who set me an example. Having lived with *parkrun* since its inception, and seen the company set up home in her back garden, she stepped back from her nursing role and joined the team. It was the perfect fit. She understood everything from the guiding principles to the inner workings, and like everyone else could get stuck in wherever it was needed. While she supported Anita in helping to establish new events in the south of England and Wales, which saw them both on the road for long periods, I also employed someone to cover the north of the country and Scotland. We also had *parkrun*s preparing to start in Northern Ireland, and so it was beginning to feel like a nationwide venture. We were making a name for ourselves as an upstart running initiative with social aims, one that played out every Saturday morning with crowds of runners gathering in parks across the four nations. Inevitably, that opened up more opportunities to forge financial partnerships to support what we were doing. I just needed the time to pursue them.

As I saw the situation, I could carry on doing things piecemeal for *parkrun* and risk the venture suffering, or give it my full attention to push for financial backing and the growth I considered to be vital. I knew that if *parkrun* was to be accessible to all then it had to be available in as many communities as possible. I just couldn't do that without putting my heart and soul into it. In 2010, I knew that it was time for me make *parkrun* my full-time occupation. The drop in salary would hurt. It certainly meant I couldn't keep injecting my own money into it. All I could do was tell myself that I would be doing something that I loved for a living, and they say that never feels like work.

Within days of joining the *parkrun* workforce in the shed, which was admittedly just down the garden path from our kitchen door, it felt like I'd come home. We were doing something innovative, facing a future that was both uncertain but hugely exciting, and that brought us all together. With the time I had been craving to commit to the venture, I set about retooling the registration and results system for growth. By the end of 2010, we had increased the number of events taking place in the UK to fifty-three. As for registered participants, the *parkrun* community had grown to become more than 100,000 strong.

Like the rest of my team, I had to wear many hats. While I was comfortable around coding, increasingly I found myself in new and strange environments as a fundraiser. I wasn't schooled in the intricacies of negotiating partnerships with commercial or government bodies. I had to learn on the fly. Very quickly, I realized that my passion for *parkrun* was perhaps more immediate than my business acumen. From a commercial perspective, I was well aware my push for growth could be interpreted as prioritizing supply over demand. While some saw that as naive, I considered it to be the definition of success for *parkrun*. I had set up Bushy Park Time Trial with no concern for the numbers that attended. I just had to be patient and believe in what I was doing. What mattered was that word spread of its existence, every Saturday morning at nine o'clock without fail. People would come in their own time, enjoy being active in good company, and that's how connections were made. The same approach had applied to the second time trial at Wimbledon Common and beyond. Essentially we would empower people to start their own events, in places that meant something to them. It didn't matter whether a dozen participants showed up or several hundred. Like a post office branch, the local pub or convenience store, *parkrun* existed to serve the community in immeasurable ways. And if financial constraints meant we couldn't provide the opportunity for an event to be established, we would have failed.

Inevitably, my pitch would often be delivered to people in charge of budgets that required some kind of measurable return. Watching *Dragon's Den* on television one evening, I briefly entertained the idea of visiting the lair to seek investment in *parkrun*. I was confident that I would command attention by describing a business that aimed to encourage communities to get active, backed up by impressive attendance figures. I just knew full well that when I dropped in that I had no intention of profiting from the venture I would be laughed back into the lift. Even if my desire to make a social difference chimed with a dragon, I recognized why they – or any successful business player, as I would find out face to face – would inevitably suggest that I risked over-reaching in my belief that creating something with purpose would attract people for all the right reasons. There were no focus groups to assess likely numbers before committing to a new event. It all came down to my faith in the power of community.

'I'm sorry, Paul, but this is mad! If you think this is how running events work then you're out of your tree!'

A former 10,000-metre world-record holder, who had gone on to become the race director of the London Marathon, David Bedford, could be regarded as running royalty. He had a reputation for being brutally direct but his opinion also mattered. At a meeting where I had pitched *parkrun* to the race organizers, with a view to securing financial backing, his response told me I faced an uphill battle. In many ways I understood his reasoning. In purely commercial terms, I was focused on supply over demand in the belief that the latter would evolve over time. In addition, I was suggesting that most people in my market for this crazy weekly event didn't consider themselves to be runners at all.

Faced with an experienced, influential figure such as Bedford, all I could do was speak from the heart. Which I chose to do after the meeting concluded when I suggested that we go for a drink.

'Think of running in this country as a pyramid,' I suggested, hoping that a more informal setting would help me to express myself. 'At the pinnacle, you have the professional athletes and world champions. The running clubs support that, and on the next level down you have the enthusiastic amateurs who run a couple of times a week or train hard for a once-in-a-lifetime London Marathon.'

Bedford sipped his pint, listening intently.

'Go on.'

'*Parkrun* sits at the foot of the pyramid,' I said. 'We're the foundation level, where people come to be active, and make a difference to their lives. The vast majority might run 5K once a week to stay in shape, or because it helps them to feel good, but among the thousands who take part every Saturday and switch onto running as a way of life there could well be tomorrow's Olympic gold medallist.'

Now I had his full attention. Even before I'd finished speaking, I could see David Bedford visualizing what I was setting out for him. We were a nursery school for running,

I suggested, and the only way to discover that talent was by opening the doors to as many people as possible.

By the time we'd finished our drinks, I had secured investment from the London Marathon to the tune of £50,000. David Bedford had placed a great deal of trust in me, and I left determined to deliver on the *parkrun* vision. Like so many individuals and organizations I met in that time, inviting them to join us in making it happen, Bedford recognized that a small investment could bring all manner of different returns.

With David Bedford on board, he even secured an opportunity that had been previously denied to us by persuading the City of London Corporation to allow us to start a *parkrun* on Hampstead Heath. In keeping with a professional athlete of his stature, having considered all the pathways in the park, Bedford even established what he believed to be the optimal course. He practically measured it to the millimetre, which rather showed me up after the redesign at Bushy Park to accommodate the rising numbers uncovered the fact that my initial circuit had been thirty metres short. Had *parkrun* been an event that participants paid to enter, this kind of amateur fumble on my part would have been unacceptable. Instead, *parkrun* had become something that belonged to the community. Together, we learned to make it work for everyone – even if I did receive a ribbing for my measuring skills – and then grow it across England, Scotland, Wales and Northern Ireland in a way that brought out the best in us all.

25

BEYOND BORDERS

In the same year that I invited runners to join me in Bushy Park one Saturday morning, Mark Zuckerburg had started the first online social network. Like Facebook, *parkrun* sought to connect people. It's just we encouraged them to do so by getting out and being active.

It was a comparison I often heard. At a time when we were striving to make it as simple as possible for people to start a *parkrun* in their own communities, however, I saw more similarities in another online phenomenon: Wikipedia.

Like *parkrun*, the free, collaborative online encyclopaedia was community driven. Founded by Jimmy Wales, a former options trader turned entrepreneur from Chicago, the resource was open to users who wished to create, edit and update their own entry. Wikipedia provided the tools for users to assemble a page on any subject under the sun, which was then monitored and maintained by a global community of volunteers.

With *parkrun*, we had built a very similar model. Anyone could start an event. We just supported them with the framework and resources they needed to get it up and running and then make it sustainable. Crispy even created a *parkrun* Wiki. It was designed as a resource for event teams and their volunteers, and provided practical advice on everything from accessibility guidelines to first-timer briefings, as well as resolving common problems when it came to processing results. Our aim was to empower people to start their own *parkrun* while acknowledging that as members of their community only they knew how to bring out the best in that event. The course design was a case in point. The event team was free to propose what they believed to be the most appropriate route for the location and just submit it for approval. In addition, every run director brought their own touch to the briefing, and that was something we actively encouraged. All we asked was that they addressed certain key points to comply with our insurance and encourage the volunteer culture to thrive.

As a result, just as every Wikipedia page is unique in terms of content, each *parkrun* event acquired its own character. In both cases, the structure behind it was the same across the board. Every *parkrun* had the same volunteer structure, from timekeepers to marshals and finish token dispensers, and started on the hour. People knew what to expect whatever their involvement in the event. What differed from one *parkrun* to the next was its personality, and that was down to the people.

This approach was key to growth, I believed. It provided

independence, ownership and encouraged responsibility, but ultimately every *parkrun* event came under the same umbrella. Which could be wide enough, I came to realize, to accommodate international events.

In 2007, we received a request from a country to a start an event that I couldn't ignore. A team of *parkrun* enthusiasts in Zimbabwe contacted me, expressing an interest in establishing a free, weekly, timed 5K in a suburb of the capital, Harare. While it resonated with me for personal reasons, as the place where I had been born, my first instinct was that it might be a step too far at a time when we were only just beginning to grow as an initiative. It was one thing to start an event across the country, but quite another halfway around the world.

Then I paused to think about what would be involved, and quickly came to the conclusion that distance was immaterial. What mattered was that the individuals who had stepped up to start an event came from that local community. As with any other new course, we provided the tools and enabled them to set up a *parkrun* that connected with the people it served. On that basis alone, Zimbabwe became the first country outside the UK to join the *parkrun* family. In establishing Rolf Valley *parkrun*, I was so proud of what that team achieved in a short space of time. They'd had to work through a bureaucratic maze, with no precedent in the country for what they were trying to do. Much like the story of Bushy Park, the early events saw a small, but enthusiastic turn out, and as word spread so the numbers grew. Sadly, political turmoil and unrest in the country forced the event to close several years later. While it didn't last for long, it burned brightly enough to show me that in *parkrun* we had something that could ignite around the world. Even so, I didn't set out a grand vision for world domination. I was too busy focusing on growth within the UK for one thing. More immediately, people were visiting *parkruns* in the UK who had some connection with other countries, and felt inspired to start events themselves.

On the European mainland, Denmark was first off the blocks. This was down to the pioneering work of British ex-pat and Copenhagen resident, Jonathan Sydenham. On his visits home, he had become a familiar parkrunner at Wimbledon Common as well as Brighton and Hove. When he approached me about the possibility of starting the first ever Scandinavian event, Jonathan's enthusiasm for sharing *parkrun* with his adopted country reminded me of how I could come across to others. By 2011, thanks to his efforts, Denmark boasted three events.

Back in the UK, as social media evolved to amplify word of mouth, *parkrun*'s steady growth tipped towards something altogether more exponential. Approaching 2012, we had close to one hundred events in England, Scotland and Wales, with almost 15,000 weekly participants. Every Saturday the number of people who joined us continued to climb, as did public awareness. As Denmark established what would become a popular home for *parkrun*, so other countries came on board.

Tim Oberg, an Australian living in London – and another Wimbledon Common regular – returned home with a vision for *parkrun* Down Under. Tim contacted us to see if we would support him despite being more than 10,000 miles away. By April 2012, largely thanks to a substantial upgrade to the registration and results system, we had the capacity to respond swiftly and positively to such interest both at home and around the world. There was no need for me to travel out each time and oversee the set-up. Internet technology allowed us to communicate closely with new teams anywhere in the world and bring them up to speed. At the same time, they had an inherent understanding of their own communities. Their insight, passion and commitment assured me that each new event was in good hands. As a result, that same month in Australia saw Main Beach *parkrun* on the Gold Coast go live. Brisbane followed shortly afterwards, with events in Melbourne and Sydney joining the *parkrun* map within the year.

Just as the lines representing growth and participation in the UK began to steepen considerably, so it seemed to draw the fledgling international lines in the same direction.

After the successful start of a single event in New Zealand, I knew exactly who I could entrust there to nurture *parkrun* in the country. On our surprise visit to Noel DeCharmoy on his fiftieth birthday, and as a time trial veteran from our running days in Johannesburg, he had been very interested to hear about my time trial in Bushy Park. When I contacted him to ask if he would like to lead the way in growing the event in New Zealand, I found Noel had been closely following *parkrun*'s progress. With my old friend on board, and just as I had seen in Denmark, he showed me that enthusiasm for a communal 5K run extended beyond borders. Thanks to the couple's tireless work, something replicated by many others around the world as countries joined the *parkrun* family, New Zealand would go on to host more than thirty weekly events to date.

As events continued to spring up, from Poland to Ireland and an early foray into the USA, I was keen to share the passion for *parkrun* with one country in particular. Since starting my new life in the UK, South Africa had been through a transformation. With apartheid dismantled, a new society had emerged determined to learn lessons from the past and look to the future. At the same time, divisions remained. Economic equalities persisted, largely along racial lines. Having seen how *parkrun* could be a great leveller, bringing everyone together no matter what their background or circumstance, I felt strongly that it could be a force for good in the place I once called home.

I also knew exactly who possessed the passion, principles and drive to lead the way in delivering that dream.

I hadn't spoken to Bruce Fordyce since the eighties, when I'd been part of his support team for the Comrades Marathon. As well as securing a reputation as one of the country's most celebrated distance runners, Bruce had been a prominent anti-apartheid activist. He was a proud countryman who continued to use his platform to seek bridges across so many divides. In early 2011 when I heard that he was visiting the UK, primarily to give a talk at Reading University about his experiences as a nine-times Comrades winner, I decided that I should go along with a view to reintroducing myself. As a reflection of his role in running history, the theatre was packed. With Bruce in conversation about his career on stage, entertaining everyone on a Friday evening, I listened to amazing stories that brought back memories from my life as a young runner. It reminded me just what an influence this man had been in showing me how determination could pay off. Afterwards, as people pressed around Bruce in the bar for a chat or an autograph, I managed to catch his attention.

'I don't know if you remember me?' I said awkwardly, aware that two decades had passed since our paths had last crossed.

Bruce registered my introduction. He paused for a beat and then grinned.

'Paul!' he beamed, and turned my handshake into an embrace.

That evening, as we caught up on each other's lives, Bruce listened with interest as I told him about my initial time trial that had turned into something much bigger than I had imagined. He hadn't heard of *parkrun*, which was no surprise to me as post-apartheid South Africa hadn't fully shaken off its insular spirit, but when I talked about the impact on communities I knew I had his full attention. During his short trip to the UK, Bruce was staying with his sister who lived in London. When he told me he would be travelling back there that evening, I realized I might have an opportunity for Bruce to experience for himself what *parkrun* could offer.

'Why don't you join me in Bushy Park tomorrow morning at nine?' I suggested. For a moment, I thought I might have trapped him into something he didn't have time to do.

'I'd never turn down a chance to go for a run,' he said instead, and arranged to meet me there.

The next morning, as people began to congregate ahead of the start, I prepared myself for the possibility that he might not turn up. Bruce and his wife, Gill, had a busy agenda before flying home. When they both found me in the crowd, however, dressed in their running gear, I just knew that it was time to let the event take over. Even in middle age, Bruce could still be a competitive runner. I half expected him to lead the way, and though he set a decent pace I could tell that he was more interested in the experience than achieving a target time.

On filing through the finishing funnel, a little breathless but beaming, Bruce Fordyce understood why I had said this was not a race but a community gathering.

'You're onto something!' he said on spotting me, and I knew he wasn't just talking about the run but everything else that the event had to offer.

I watched him join the growing throng of finishers, people of every age and ability chatting happily, and felt quite sure that he had just taken the first step towards bringing *parkrun* to a country that could benefit from events in both cities and townships.

Later that year, Bruce and the team he had assembled launched South Africa's first *parkrun* in Delta Park, Johannesburg. I had no doubt that the country's strong running culture would embrace the concept, but Bruce went the extra mile in encouraging a diversity of participants. He focused on establishing events in economically deprived areas, and emphasized inclusion and health. In particular, Bruce welcomed walkers as much as runners. It meant people got involved who might otherwise have been deterred, and that took *parkrun* to another level in terms of activity for all. By 2013, *parkrun* had established 20 events nationwide. By 2020, that number would surpass 200, with up to 70,000 people taking part each week. Thanks to the early efforts of Bruce Fordyce, and the values he has always represented, South Africa would become one of the largest *parkrun* communities outside the UK.

To date, *parkrun* is thriving in over twenty-five countries, from Norway to Namibia, and Germany to Japan, Poland and Canada. The USA is beginning to discover the magic that can be had from a free, weekly 5K, with events springing up from Alabama to Wisconsin. There are always challenges in every country, of course. Sometimes there are cultural issues. In America jogging has long been considered to be a solitary activity. That view is changing as people switch onto the joys of running or walking together, and in some ways *parkrun* USA is leading the way. Elsewhere, we've faced bureaucratic hurdles. In France, red tape has led us with regret to suspend events there. Despite the current position of the authorities, insisting that all participants obtain medical certificates, I still hope that as *parkrun* grows in other countries it will demonstrate that we're pursuing the same aim: an active, positive and connected society.

When I spin a virtual globe on my computer screen, with 2,300 pins representing the current number of *parkrun* events around the world, each one represents to me a community effort to share the same vision. Recently, I travelled to Lithuania to meet a quietly spoken, humble man with huge enthusiasm for starting *parkrun* in his country. Like so many event organizers, Alexandr Sorokin recognized the benefits that it could bring to his community near the centre of the capital, Vilnius. Working together, so that Alexandr and his team could gain first-hand experience before the official launch, we staged a test run in the beautiful grounds of Vingis Park. As a small field shuttled around the course he had carefully marked out, my new friend was focused solely on how to make the event as accessible as possible. He offered nothing but smiles and encouragement from the first finisher to the last, and engaged with his volunteers throughout.

'Do you run much?' I asked him at one point.

'A little,' he said shyly, but in a way that told me he was passionate about it.

Afterwards, over coffee and delicious cake at a cafe outside the park, I fell into conversation with another member of the team.

'Alexandr is a multiple world record holder for long distance running,' she told me, having overheard our earlier chat. 'He's the fastest man in history to run 100 miles in 10 hours and 51 minutes, but he'd never tell you that himself.'

Across the floor of the cafe, I set eyes on this quiet, unassuming superhuman, and understood exactly why he had been drawn to *parkrun*.

'We all have to start somewhere,' I said.

26

CHANGES & CHALLENGES

Had the Ghost of *parkrun* Future visited me the night before the first time trial at Bushy Park, I would have done things very differently. When I arrived in the car park on that Saturday morning in 2004, I had brought with me fifty washers with numbers printed on them. Even then I knew full well that it would take time before I got the chance to hand them all out at the finish line.

While I was prepared for nobody to show up, thirteen runners put my system to the test. All I wanted to do was produce a set of results so that each participant could see their time and position. They could compare themselves to others in the field if they wished, which was one of my aims at the time, or run it another week and go into competition with themselves. That was about the extent of my ambition. While my desire to bring people together has remained the same, it didn't come close to where *parkrun* is today. As a consequence, over the last twenty-one years we've had to evolve rapidly when required in order to stay one step ahead of everything from demand to technology.

It's fair to say that most successful endeavours started from a very different place. Like Zuckerberg in his student digs, coding a programme to connect his fellow students on campus, I didn't draw up a grand plan to create a global community. I might have played a small role in *parkrun*'s evolution, but ultimately it's been a collective effort by a committed organization and a community that has grown to millions who participate every week. We've had to adapt or dig deep to overcome obstacles, none of which I ever imagined I'd encounter when I started. There have been times when it felt like an uphill struggle, or we faced an unexpected trip hazard. In every case, it's been a question of keeping our eyes and ears open, continuing to put one foot in front of the other, and believing that the outcome will always reward the effort.

After an institutionalized upbringing, and a career working with systems, I tend to look at life in terms of the processes behind it. I appreciate that my background means I can get unusually excited about the mechanics of how things work. It's not for everyone, of course. Generally, what matters to people is the outcome. When it comes to *parkrun*, the rewards for each participant go far beyond anything I ever foresaw. Whatever their reasons for showing up, it's also a feelgood moment at the end of each week. As much as I've always loved to hear the stories about what people get out of *parkrun*, I can never lose sight of the process that went into making it happen.

Before the very first event in Bushy Park, my aim was to create something with simplicity at its heart. Anyone could take part and then feature in the results that followed. I didn't just want to make it easy for participants, but for me too.

Over time, that proved to be the hardest part.

In those early years, as the number of participants and events grew steadily but slowly, I found the washer system coped just fine. Eventually, however, the demand for washers exceeded my enthusiasm for hand-punching numbers into each one. I went online and sourced a supply of individually numbered aluminium tags from the USA Forestry Commission. While the tags were intended for use in identifying sapling trees, I found they did the same job as the steel washers in tracking finishing positions, but also spared my patio flagstones from further risk of cracks. During this time, use of barcodes became more sophisticated and prevalent in everyday life, from grocery shopping to ticket authentication. Critically for me, they also became more affordable. In 2009, as part of the results system upgrade, Crispy and I rolled out a new feature that assigned a unique barcode to each participant as well as to a new kind of finish token designed just for *parkrun*. With volunteers on hand to scan every individual's personal barcode and finish token, effectively linking the two for that event, the data could be transferred to a computer where the results would take shape at the touch of a button. Once we issued a laptop to each event team, coffee and cake became a whole lot more productive.

As part of the online registration process, newcomers simply had to print out their barcode and take it with them to an event. It really was as easy as that. By effectively going digital, we had also prepared *parkrun* for the steep growth curve that followed.

Throughout the history of *parkrun*, and having worked with computers throughout my career, I'd always aimed to embrace technology as a means of making things easier. In 2004, most people had email addresses and access to dial-up internet, and I seized on it as a way to deliver results. Having come up with the *parkrun* name, Stuart Lodge played another pivotal role by helping me create a website capable of sharing current and past results for each event. As the software became more sophisticated, I added features like age categories, the number of times an individual had volunteered or run, and any club affiliation. I even incorporated a measure that calculated a runner's performance as a percentage of the best possible time for their age and gender. As fairness was a value dear to me, age grading helped to standardize the results for each event and make performances more comparable across the field. Starting with a website that was little more than a digital flyer, we now have a resource that allows people to drill into their data or access event details anywhere in the world.

For me, perhaps the most significant change in *parkrun*'s evolution has been the average finishing time. Over the course of twenty-one years, it's become slower. This may seem counterintuitive to some, but I see it as a sign that *parkrun* is achieving its aims.

At the very first time trial, thirteen individuals lined up

wearing athletics shorts or Lycra leggings, poised to start their sports watches. Many wore club vests, but not everybody. Some considered themselves to be casual runners, but even then the last one over the line finished in under thirty minutes, which could be considered relatively quick. Had anyone finished in double that time, I would have taken it in my stride. My event was always open to anyone, after all. I had just failed to consider that it would draw people who sometimes didn't even think of themselves as runners at all. It was a happy discovery. As young and old began to join, the scope of ability broadened. Some came who were recovering from injury, illnesses or operations. Others saw it as a chance to get out of the house and enjoy some fresh air or found it helped with managing mental health conditions. People incorporated *parkrun* into a weight loss routine, or pushed buggies around the course with infants strapped in for the ride. Some of those sleep-deprived new parents proved to be formidable runners, too. Even today, should you find yourself overtaken by a parent and baby duo on two feet and four wheels then you should consider yourself to have been 'prammed'.

As this glorious collective took shape over the years, representing different backgrounds, abilities and objectives, so that average finishing time began to grow a little longer. Admittedly, it masks the fact that light-footed runners have always counted among this number. Indeed, at Edinburgh *parkrun* in 2023, the British Olympian, Andy Butchart, set the fastest recorded time of 13 minutes and 45 seconds. It's an incredible achievement, and stands alongside the efforts of the last person over the line that morning who finished in just over 51 minutes as part of an NHS couch to 5K programme. While Nick Griggs would take Andy's record by a second just one year later at Belfast Victoria *parkrun*, I'm delighted that some finishing times now tip over an hour. From the front of the field to the back, everyone is sharing in the same activity, and achieving something extraordinary. When it comes to the nation's health, that has to be a change for good.

For all the advances that we strived to make, of course, *parkrun* has encountered some bumps along the way. Right from the start, I have made mistakes. Sure enough, it took time for the teasing to stop when it was discovered that the first course I established at Bushy Park measured short. What's key to me is that screw-ups like this are something we learn from. While the new course was extended to hit the correct distance, I can look back on several other significant events as episodes that challenged us but which ultimately improved the *parkrun* experience.

Inevitably, much of it comes down to money. Having started as a personally funded project, which then became a not-for-profit organization, *parkrun* has had to take great care in developing relationships with commercial partners in a way that respects our independence. Having enjoyed lasting relationships with companies such as Nike, Lucozade Sport, Vitality, Sweatshop, Adidas, Intersport, Co-op and Brooks, we have broadly maintained our aims. I can also count Hutchison among that number. Having shown me such understanding and flexibility when what was supposed to be a personal project began to impact on my time as a consultant, my former client went on to help support *parkrun* by providing us with modems for the event team laptops.

In order to maintain stability as an organization, it's been important to nurture a diverse family of backers that align with *parkrun*'s values. It's not easy to strike the right balance. We certainly stumbled when we briefly brought on board an egg company whose methods of production sparked protests across the community. In many ways, it was a stark reminder that *parkrun* belongs to the people, who made it clear such a partnership was out of step with our values. I can be stubborn about many things in life, but equally when I'm wrong then the only way forward is through humility and a willingness to do better.

In any pioneering venture, there is no road map. We're not following a well-trodden path. We're finding our own way. Sometimes, that means we make wrong turns. It can also lead to unexpected diversions that call into question where we're going but ultimately focus attention on our destination.

In 2017, the local council in Stoke Gifford near Bristol announced that it intended to charge the Little Stoke *parkrun* for using the park grounds. Councillors argued that the event placed additional strain on public resources and justified a fee. I was surprised by their stand. On the whole, local councils had always been generous and accommodating in allowing us to stage events in parks and public places. They recognized the value to the community and together we've formed lasting relationships. If issues arose, which were commonly around subjects like public safety or parking, we addressed them privately and constructively.

In this case, the local parish council in Stoke Gifford issued a press release. By adopting a position that threatened to put an end to an event unless *parkrun* agreed to pay a fee, the episode made national headlines.

While I questioned that any *parkrun* caused tangible wear and tear, I was heartened that the outcry didn't just come from parkrunners but the wider running community. In operating a free not-for-profit event to promote health and inclusivity, we rejected the council's position. Health advocates and even UK government officials spoke out against the fee. At the same time, I knew that other councils were awaiting the outcome to review their position. Had we folded, it would have set a precedent and made *parkrun* unsustainable. Ultimately, we took the decision to close Little Stoke *parkrun* rather than pay to put on the event. It was a sad day, but one that highlighted the importance of public spaces for community health initiatives and solidified support for *parkrun*'s free model across the UK.

I have always believed that within every obstacle is an opportunity waiting to emerge. Sometimes that can be hard to appreciate, and there have been moments in the history of *parkrun* when I have sensed a pull in the wrong direction or felt let down by people in a position of trust. In every case, openness and honesty had led to positive resolutions, even if that conversation can be painful or give rise to strong feelings. In a recent bid to tighten our focus on community, health and inclusivity, *parkrun* removed several categories of statistics from the website. We retired the Fastest 500 feature for each course, as well as age and gender category records. The aim was to shift the emphasis away from speed and performance and to encourage participation and personal enjoyment, especially for newcomers who might feel intimidated by what could be construed as a competitive atmosphere.

Inevitably, the decision sparked heated debate among the *parkrun* community.

Many regular participants considered these statistics as personal milestones and motivational tools. Runners who enjoy tracking progress over time expressed disappointment. In some quarters it was seen as a loss of community history and tradition, while limiting transparency and accountability. In particular, many reasoned that taking away gender-based records discouraged female athletes from achieving their goals. Some also viewed the removal of particular stats as a way for *parkrun* to sidestep calls for the creation of a category for transgender participants.

I heard every viewpoint. I listened to the feedback and took it all on board. I also registered the strength of feeling throughout, particularly from those who see gender-based and age-category records as valuable motivators. In response, I began by making it quite clear that the decision to implement the changes was part of a long-term strategy, and in no way a response to the debate around transgender participants. We had been planning to remove the stats in question for years, and though in hindsight we could have communicated our reasons more clearly I stand by the changes we made. I recognize the sensitivities surrounding the subject, and welcome the conversation around it as a listening and learning experience, but my priority is inclusivity for all. Age, gender and ability all have their place, of course, and the fact is many of those statistics that have been removed are still available to participants from their profile pages. They've just been repositioned to celebrate individual achievements rather than by a category comparison that will never work for everyone.

Ultimately, *parkrun* is a broad church that aims to bring people together through the shared aims of getting active and having fun. I absolutely agree that competition can be a healthy thing. There's a joy to be had from seeing runners side by side in a sprint for the finishing funnel, but at *parkrun* that's between them. Collectively, I just hope that we can move forward with the same mutual respect for everyone that I see on the course every Saturday morning, and continue to bring out the best in each other.

27

A LITTLE BIT OF SUNSHINE

Over the course of twenty years, *parkrun* has welcomed runners of all ages. With children, parents and grandkids in the mix, it's not uncommon to find four generations taking part in a single event. Since 2004, some early adopters of the weekly time trial now bring children of their own. The Russell family are my favourite example, simply because I've known them since the start. Young James was one of the thirteen pioneers who lined up for the first Bushy Park Time Trial, followed soon afterwards by his brother, Grant. The brothers are now on their journey from their 500th milestone t-shirt to their 1000th, and while James's kids have some way to go they're just as enthusiastic. They've always known *parkrun*, starting out as pushchair occupants and then running with their parents. Nor are they unique. Across the *parkrun* community, young people following in the footsteps of their parents or guardians, siblings or friends, have embraced something that's increasingly off limits to them in the modern world, and that's the chance to get active together.

In the beginning, my focus was on setting down roots for Bushy Park Time Trial so that it could grow. I was quite happy when people brought along their children to run with them. I held the view that it was the responsibility of the parents to be sure they were safe and having fun, and that's exactly how it shaped up over the years. Often, a participant would show up with a young family in tow to spectate. Those kids would invariably decide that running around the course was perhaps the more exciting option and make overtures to join in next time. Naturally, it only takes the sight of a couple of younger participants to encourage more to follow. When buggies joined the mix, along with grandparents, it just strengthened my growing conviction that what we had here was something for all.

While it was great to see youngsters taking part in those early years, I also heard people question if five kilometres was too far for some. We already asked that children who took part on foot should be aged four or over, with anyone under eleven in the company of a responsible adult. At the same time, I recognized that age is not a measure of ability at any time of life. Some kids took on the time trial with speed and grace while others sauntered along and stopped to inspect bugs and flowers.

With this in mind, Bushy sports coach and occupational therapist, Paul Graham, approached me to suggest a version of *parkrun* that would give ownership to children and young people. With a course measuring two kilometres, he reasoned that the distance would be in line with *parkrun*'s values of making it accessible to all. As someone who supported children with learning difficulties, and mindful of my own feeling of freedom on running a lap of the playing field at school for the very first time, Paul set out a compelling case. There would be no pressure on kids to run, and should they choose to walk the course it would still only take a maximum of half an hour. I recognized the benefits. I could also see potential problems, which came down to safeguarding. We had a duty of care, after all, but as our conversation continued it became clear that parents or guardians would be key to the success of such an event. They would be present, after all, which created a pool of volunteers with a vested interest in making it a success.

It was early in 2010. We had just launched our thirtieth *parkrun* event, and focused on expanding at full tilt as more volunteer teams established events in their communities. Given Paul's expertise and enthusiasm for starting an event at Bushy Park for children and young adults, I was happy to let him lead the way while providing him with all the support he needed.

The first junior *parkrun*, as we called it, was held in April. As a trial, we decided to run it on the first Sunday of each month. Recognizing that busy parents would benefit from the extra hour shepherding their kids out of the house and into the park, we settled on a 10 a.m. start. With marshals stationed around the course so that no young participant was ever out of eye shot, and plenty of parents accompanying kids whose confidence would take some time to grow, Paul Graham started a bespoke version of *parkrun* for anyone aged between four and fourteen years old. Like our inaugural junior *parkrun* director, along with a small army of volunteers, I put on my high-vis tabard in my role as token scanner and hoped the event would go off without a hitch.

The good news was that every child was kept safe and happy from start to finish. The tweaked system we had established to collect results also worked wonders. Paul and his team did a terrific job in making the first junior *parkrun* a success, even if it did feel like controlled chaos at times.

'Great run . . . keep going . . . loving the racing car noises . . . this way!'

In dealing with so many children, we soon learned that herding cats would have been an easier task. The kids were lovely. They brought bags of enthusiasm with them, even if many didn't have a clue what was going on. Through their eyes, however, the experience was *joyful*; a chance to walk, jog, run or skip around the course with new friends, laughing and chattering under the watchful eye of an occupational therapist who showed no sign of wishing that he was at home with the Sunday papers. The true test came just after the finishing funnel, where participants presented their personal barcode and finishing token to me – the volunteer with the scanner – so the results can be registered and compiled.

I had one job that morning, which immediately presented itself with all manner of complications, as excited children sought to trade their tokens like collectible cards or even bite them to see how they tasted. It was bedlam, but also brilliant fun for everyone. To be fair to the kids, the system was completely new to them. They also proved to be naturally fast learners. As both participants and volunteers gained experience from one month to the next, so it became quite clear to me that junior *parkrun* was here to stay.

In the year or so that followed, a handful of other established *parkrun* events adopted the model of staging a junior *parkrun* on Sunday. With a responsible adult in tow, children aged four and over continued to be welcome to take part in the Saturday events. It's just now they had an additional event that they could call their own. Around that time, I had the pleasure of meeting the acclaimed triathlete and four-times ironman world champion, Chrissie Wellington. Approaching retirement from the sport, Chrissie was looking for a new challenge. In particular, she was interested in doing something meaningful that would make a difference to the next generation. When I outlined the baby steps we had taken to creating an event for younger participants, she struck me as the right person to grow and develop the initiative.

Since 2013, when we welcomed Chrissie Wellington into the organization, junior *parkrun* has grown from four monthly events in the UK to more than 425 worldwide, with the majority taking place every Sunday. Over the course of fifteen years, nearly half a million four- to fourteen-year-olds have taken part in an event that puts safeguarding first and provides an opportunity for everyone involved to have a great time. Many are now adults who continue to enjoy active lives. I've no doubt that this formative experience has had a positive impact. I only have to consider those junior *parkrun* graduates who so often become regulars at the Saturday 5K to appreciate it has made a difference. For them and many others, running shouldn't just be something that they're made to do at school. It's an intrinsic and often highly social part of life that feels as natural as breathing, while we all recognize the wider benefits in terms of physical and mental wellbeing. In time, I sincerely hope that junior *parkrun* contributes to a generational change to the way we live our lives.

Week after week, I see kids gain confidence in themselves and in what is possible for them to achieve. It's about taking on a challenge with support from family, volunteers and peers, and feeling rewarded in a social setting that can see them step up in other ways. Many young regulars take on volunteer roles themselves, and often it's the quieter ones that shine. Hosting the warm-up session is a case in point. It's something tailor-made for the Sunday events, and the one role that sees me staring at the ground if the volunteer co-ordinator is looking for an adult to fill the role. Leading the way with star jumps is just not for me, and yet all too often it's the shy junior parkrunner who's taken part in plenty that offers to lead the way. Why? Because they're among friends in a safe and familiar environment, and it's a chance for them to step up on their path to adulthood. Just recently, at a Saturday *parkrun*, a man introduced himself to me as the father of the first finisher.

'My son took part in junior *parkrun* for years, and it did wonders for his self-esteem.' He nodded towards a young man, a little puffed and red in the face, who was chatting cheerily with a volunteer. 'He discovered that with hard work and the right support he could achieve something, and that transformed his life.'

The great thing about *parkrun*'s evolution is that the best ideas have come from participants. In the same way that Paul Graham identified a way to make a difference to the lives of children, so Shane Spencer approached us in late 2016 with a proposal for *parkrun* to play a positive role in the welfare and rehabilitation of prisoners.

A gym manager at HMP Haverigg in Cumbria, and enthusiastic parkrunner, Shane believed that establishing an event for inmates within prison walls would bring the same physical and mental benefits to inmates as it did to communities around the world. Like junior *parkrun*, it wasn't something I had ever considered. In the same way, I could see how it would bring something positive to the lives of people who could perhaps most benefit from it.

An initiative led by Chrissie Wellington, working alongside HM Prison and Probation Service, the first *parkrun* in a custodial facility took place six months later at HMP Haverigg. Known as Black Combe *parkrun*, which is the name of a prominent hill that overlooks the prison grounds, the event was set up by Shane Spencer and a volunteer team comprising of both prison staff and inmates. Over the course of eight loops of the prison yard, and to the sound of the usual banter and encouragement, twenty-four participants enjoyed the same positive experience as millions of people at *parkrun* events around the world. Some ran, others walked and plenty talked and laughed. Afterwards, in the prison sports hall, volunteers, runners and walkers even had a chance to enjoy a chat over tea and coffee.

Behind the scenes, it had been a complex undertaking that both Chrissie and Shane handled with sensitivity and a shared sense of purpose. Taking place in a closed facility, vetted inmates could participate by invitation only. Immediately, it became a driver for good behaviour. In his dual role as gym manager and event director, Shane encouraged inmates to take part whom he believed would most benefit from the experience. He approached those who didn't work out or struggled with self-esteem issues, and just asked them to give it a chance.

After the success of the first event, with results posted on a noticeboard along with the opportunity to sign up to volunteer at future events, Black Combe *parkrun* swiftly became a regular high point for the Haverigg prison community. Prison exercise is nothing new, of course, but this was far from a monotonous, isolating or intimidating experience. Shane's *parkrun* built positive relationships between inmates and staff, promoted health and wellbeing on being outdoors, while ultimately forging a sense of purpose on the path towards rehabilitation.

In some ways, the *parkrun* model seemed purpose-built to bring out the best in a custodial community. Just as it had taken off in the outside world, so other prisons learned about the success of Black Combe *parkrun* and sought to replicate it for themselves. Today, over twenty-five *parkrun*s have been established in correctional facilities across the UK, Ireland and Australia, including women's prisons and young offenders institutes. Collectively, they've hosted over 3,500 events with over 70,000 walks or runs completed by 11,500 participants. That has to be a force for good, and another branch on the *parkrun* tree that I hope will continue to flourish.

While a *parkrun* in a prison is off limits to the general public, participants are permitted to invite special guests.

Often, prison governors and staff will answer the call to lace up their trainers, as well as local community leaders or charity representatives. Kelly Holmes, in the tireless role she so kindly accepted from me some years earlier as *parkrun* ambassador, has taken part in several events, as has John McAvoy, a former armed robber, ex-prisoner turned endurance athlete and advocate for positive change through sports. John is living proof that anyone can turn their lives around, and I am so proud of his passionate support for *parkrun* in prisons.

On several occasions, I have been honoured with an invitation to participate at events in both male and female prisons. Everything about the events is recognisable to an outsider, from the signage to the finishing tokens and the milestone t-shirts so proudly worn by some. Even the fun, chatty and communal atmosphere is just the same as it is at any event around the world. The difference, I think, is in the impact of the value it brings to the participants. Recently, I took part in an event at a youth offenders facility. I fell in with a lad and we started talking as we walked and jogged. He told me that he felt anxious being in the prison gym environment, whereas the *parkrun* event made equals of everybody who took part. We took our time on the course, and in doing so he began to open up to me. In short, he felt a deep sense of embarrassment that his life choices had led him here. With his sentence nearing its end, he was looking forward to doing something positive with his future. While he wasn't sure what that would look like, my new friend was quite certain of one thing: *parkrun* would be a regular feature of his life on the outside.

On one level, *parkrun* can seem like an insignificant activity. It's just a run, or a walk, after all. It can mean more things for us all, of course, and yet for those who are just starting out in life, or hoping to make a fresh start, the community embracing it can provide a little bit of sunshine and a sense of belonging as they find their feet in the world.

28

PEOPLE ARE GOOD

For years, the shed at the bottom of my garden served as the operations centre for a bid to get the world up on its feet. Together with Crispy, Anita and Jo, I maximized every inch of available space so that we could all work comfortably if we happened to be there at the same time. I even commandeered the section reserved for my tools and converted it into a room for the company's computer servers.

While also bringing on board regional representatives in Leeds and Glasgow, we worked tirelessly with communities in the UK and overseas to roll out new events. Every day brought new challenges and opportunities, none of which came with a road map. Nobody had done anything like this before. We were pioneers, just like the thirteen runners who had taken part in the very first time trial – who would each receive a gold version of their personal barcode on *parkrun*'s tenth birthday in recognition of their contribution to the *parkrun* story.

For just over a decade, that little shed was home to what sometimes felt like a punk rock running organization. We were shaking up the established way of staging events by keeping participation completely free and open to all. Inevitably, as *parkrun* events began to pop up across the UK, and participant numbers climbed, commercial players began to pay attention. Through their eyes, it wasn't about community but the potential to cash in. A couple of race organizations attempted to start their own 5K events. They were slick operations that charged to participate, and quickly failed. In my opinion, the reason wasn't all down to money. As *parkrun* took off, advances in sport technology meant that timing mats became an affordable option to record finishers at the line. Participants simply wore a band with a chip that would automatically trigger sensors in the mat to record their unique ID, time and position. On paper, it was a much more efficient way to compile results than deploying a volunteer with a stopwatch and another with a barcode scanner. Our rivals figured we couldn't afford the upgrade to compete with what was no doubt a slicker process.

My view was that the use of a timing mat at *parkrun* would take away what I still consider to be the most precious part of the experience. Instead of gathering on the far side of the finish funnel to catch their breath, fall into conversation and then finally take their barcode and finish token to the volunteer with the scanner and the chance for another chat, participants at the new events simply melted away. Rather than take time to talk, laugh, cool down and unwind, they simply headed for the park exits. The timing mats allowed results to be compiled automatically, which is great for efficiency but it cost those rival events to *parkrun* in terms of community.

For this reason alone, *parkrun* employs the same process that began with the time trial in 2004. The technology might have changed – with volunteers now using apps on their phones to record times and positions – but that moment after participants finish is a truly magical and sociable time for everyone, and frankly nothing can replace it. Yes, it might be ragged and inefficient to a commercial operation, but we're not about profit but people.

Keeping *parkrun* free and open to all has been hard work. Early on, my brother, Tim, stepped up when I needed him by loaning me funds at a difficult time to keep things afloat. We've remained close, even though he returned to South Africa some time ago. When our sister, Lindsay, sadly passed away, it reminded us both of a time when neither of us could take family for granted. Over the years, *parkrun* has become just as precious to me. As an organization we've also been very fortunate in working alongside sponsorship partners who continue to share our vision. In fact, when Covid stopped the world from turning in so many ways, every single one stood by us. Their support enabled us to restart as restrictions eased at a time when the benefits of *parkrun* were more important than ever before. For all the challenges we faced, ultimately it's been hugely rewarding in seeing how *parkrun* can make a difference to individuals and communities.

Even so, there comes a time when an upstart venture must become an established organization in order to deliver its mission. For *parkrun*, having sprung out of the running scene and then evolved to welcome one and all, that moment arrived in 2015. We were hiring in order to keep up with growth, which meant the shed at the bottom of my garden could no longer contain us. Moving our headquarters down the road to Eel Pie Island, which sits between the banks of the River Thames, coincided with a more significant change within the organization. Having led a not-for-profit company for the best part of a decade, and with a number of weekly participants topping 100,000 worldwide, I felt that our wonderful community had outgrown the abilities of a computer systems guy to lead the way. The time had come, I decided, for me to hand over to others with the skills and experience to take *parkrun* to the next level.

Just over a year after we left the garden shed behind, *parkrun* became a registered UK charity. It was perhaps the most significant change in the history of the organization. After my battles to keep *parkrun* free and accessible for all, the change of status effectively enshrined our aims in a constitution. It protected its legacy as much as its future, and played a key role in persuading me to step back from leading the way. Resigning as Chief Executive, I took a seat on the board of trustees and together we embarked upon a clear mission: to make the world healthier and happier. It was an ambitious statement but one that opened up opportunities for *parkrun* to extend its reach. By effectively turning from a sports organization to a public health and wellbeing initiative, *parkrun* was in a better position to work with governments and authorities around the world in establishing events. The free, weekly format remained unchanged, but that's where the conversation started about revising the presentation of statistics to more closely align with our goals as a charity. Ultimately, providing people with every opportunity to participate remains the overarching objective.

Watching the new charity spread its wings was a proud moment for me. Today, *parkrun* employs over seventy people not just in its new office in Richmond, south-west London, but also in Australia, Japan, Ireland, the Netherlands, South Africa and Canada. At the same time, I found it difficult to adjust to an existence away from the frontline of the organization. Right from the start, it had consumed me in the most wonderful way. From the moment I saw something special evolving in the community that formed around those early events, *parkrun* had taken up all my time and energy for almost twelve years. In that period, I had learned more about myself than ever before as well as what great things can be achieved when people come together.

I knew the transition back to an ordinary life would be hard. On the upside, I had plans to spend more time with my new wife. In 2009, as a changed man from the one she had first met with all the self-doubts and commitment issues, I proposed to Jo and was delighted when she accepted. In the years since our marriage, we said goodbye to Tim the dog, who will always be remembered as my first four-legged running buddy, and welcomed Dotty into the fold, another springer spaniel who turned circles around us both and brought us nothing but joy throughout her life. Jo and I also developed a shared interest in cycling. I had recovered from the injuries that sidelined me from running, and which indirectly transformed everything for me. Having reached my mid-fifties, however, I found that riding a bike was kinder on my joints. I was also well aware that my fastest times were behind me. The dream of running a marathon in under two and a half hours was long gone, but I could still look back and be proud that I had given it my best shot. I also recognized that it had taken me on a journey that I wouldn't change for the world.

While I had stepped back from the organization, I remained a committed *parkrun* participant. As a volunteer, runner, jogger or walker, I still enjoy visiting different events with Jo to experience what the community has created. It's a chance to chat to people and, of course, enjoy the cake and coffee afterwards. Each event is unique, even if the course distance is – more or less – the same. It's defined by everything from the park or open space that hosts the course to the people who take part. Some events are huge, sprawling affairs. Bushy *parkrun* – as the original is now called – has always remained the biggest of all, with over 6,000 people taking part one Saturday in September 2024 to mark the 1000th event. Others are low-key but no less vital, and often serve economically deprived, rural or isolated communities. If just five people take part, I will support that as much as the events with numbers in quadruple figures.

Wherever we go, no matter what the location or attendance, it always feels like a special moment at the end of the week. People show up for all kinds of reasons, but ultimately we're there because it's a positive experience we can share together.

Often, Jo and I will arrive at an event where we don't

know anyone. During the week, we might have gone to the *parkrun* website and registered to volunteer, or we're there to line up at the start with everyone else after the director's briefing so we all know what to expect. Either way, as new faces we're always made to feel welcome. Like any newcomer, we quickly find ourselves chatting freely with the people around us.

In the days when *parkrun* was rising into the public consciousness, I would often be invited to make media appearances. Whether it was newspapers, websites, television or radio, I became quite evangelical about my passion for what we were doing. As a result, I unintentionally became a familiar voice and face to many, particular those who had already embraced *parkrun* as a mainstay of their communities. It meant that as *parkrun* grew bigger more people at events started to recognize me.

As someone who grew up on the edge of things, I really appreciate the sense of belonging to be found at any *parkrun* event. What I've had to get used to over the years, however, is that for a short time on a Saturday morning I can find myself in a spotlight. Generally it starts when someone approaches to politely ask for a selfie. I'm always happy to oblige, but in doing so it draws more attention and fuels word that 'the founder' is present. I always want to stress that I just played a small role in it all. I planted a seed at a time when I was struggling and wanted to be active, outdoors and social.

What I didn't realize was that so did everyone else.

A social movement is a collection of people with shared ideals and a vision for change. It doesn't have to be an uprising or revolution. Sometimes, we can all be on the same side. We just have to make it happen. I will never be comfortable with the accolades that have come from being the one who invited others to join me. For me, every single individual who ever participated in *parkrun* has played a valuable role. Without the global community that has grown up around it, I'd still be that slightly lost soul who pledged to be in the same place in the park with a stopwatch once a week.

In this view, when people come up to me at *parkrun* events, I feel that I should be thanking them.

As well as the selfies, many just want to share their stories about what *parkrun* means to them. It has been a privilege to hear so many accounts from people about how it's changed their lives. Sometimes it may not seem like much, from a chance to catch up with a friend, lose a little weight or run without feeling the pressure of a race, but it means a great deal to them. Everyone has a different experience, but in every case it's a positive one. For some, and this always leaves me lost for words, *parkrun* has become a reason for choosing to live.

I feel privileged to have heard so many accounts of the impact of *parkrun* on people. There is one that stays in mind above all others because it was the first time I realized the potential it had to make a difference. A few months after the first event at Bushy Park, a big guy approached me who had just written down his finishing number next to his name on the clipboard in the boot of my car. He had been a few times before, and the five-kilometre distance was clearly quite some undertaking for a man of his build.

'I was watching the London Marathon on TV with my

little daughter,' he said, having really just popped across to thank me. 'She prodded my tummy and said, "You're too fat to do that, Daddy," and honestly it destroyed me. I didn't want to be that kind of father, and decided to do something about it. So, that's why I've started coming here.' He paused there to mop his brow. 'One day I'm going to run that marathon.'

'That's brilliant! Your daughter must be very proud of you!'

When he didn't seem to register my response, I realized he had something else to tell me. Still catching his breath, the guy looked around as if to make sure he couldn't be overheard by the men and women milling around in club vests.

'You know, this isn't just for proper runners,' said my new friend, and then lowered his voice like he had a secret to share. 'Paul, it's for *everyone*.'

Today, I still think about that man's simple observation, and how prescient it was. I also hope he fulfilled his ambition, though I've no doubt that just getting active brought its own reward. Over twenty years on, I can look back with the benefit of hindsight and recognize what it took to make my own dream a reality. First and foremost, as human beings we can do amazing things when we're all engaged with something that feels meaningful. If there's one thing that this incredible journey constantly reminds me, it is that essentially people are good. Then there are the principles behind *parkrun*, which haven't changed since I set out to do something for the sake of my health and happiness and then realized I wasn't alone. We've had to adapt as momentum took over, but those values inform every step we take so we never stray from the path.

In my book, that's how to grow a social movement.

I'm in my mid-sixties now, and a proud grandfather. What *parkrun* has taught me is that age is no barrier when it comes to finding a purpose and sense of belonging. Anyone can set out to make a difference in their community, bring people together and transform lives – including their own – in the process. It might sound like a dream, but comes down to believing in good things and taking one step at a time. Recently, as our children had all grown up to pursue independent lives, Jo and I said goodbye to our home in London for a rural life in a village in West Sussex. We've made new friends and started exploring the countryside by bike and on foot. There, every Tuesday afternoon, I collect a lively springer spaniel from a neighbour so that he can work without the need to throw a tennis ball every ten seconds. I just love the breed; their zest for life is infectious. The dog's name is Sprint, which seems fitting, and although I no longer chase times I wish I had his boundless energy. At *parkrun*, I still pay attention when people strive for a personal best,. It's just nowadays I find talking to other people over the 5k course has become my reward. With this in mind, whenever I volunteer I often take on the recently created role of parkwalker.

In my view, this is one of the most rewarding ways to experience *parkrun*. At events in South Africa, thanks to the efforts of Bruce Fordyce and his team to make everyone welcome, there can often be more walkers than runners. With this in mind, *parkrun* introduced the role of parkwalker to demonstrate that walking is both valued and encouraged. People may choose to walk for health reasons, or in taking the first steps towards a more active lifestyle. Some might just want to be social, which is why I love wearing the blue tabard with *parkwalker* emblazoned on the back. In effect, it's a friendly face who takes on the course at a gentle stroll so that people don't feel compelled to jog or run. The parkwalker doesn't need to be last. Just available to anyone who wishes to take their time and complete the course in company.

And in doing so, this is where I hear personal stories that capture the *parkrun* spirit.

Recently, as parkwalker at my local event, I was joined by a lovely lady in her seventies along with her granddaughter. The little girl was no more than five years old, and so talkative. She told me her name, favourite dog breed – dachshunds – and the fact that she could jump really high. Within the space of a minute, in which she barely paused to draw breath, I realized she was going to leave me exhausted for quite charming reasons.

'Daddy is fast,' she declared, after her grandmother had added that the pair were seasoned parkrunners, taking part that morning, and in a constant state of friendly competition with one another, 'but Mummy is faster.'

'Well, let's find out how they did at the finish,' I said. 'But first we've got to find our way there.'

For some, five kilometres can seem like a long way. As a five-year-old, it must be hard to appreciate any distance, which is why adults are so familiar with being asked if we're nearly there yet. Under a clear blue sky, and to the sound of skylarks on the breeze, the little girl didn't once ask that question. Instead, she continued to lead both the way and the conversation. As we walked, I learned that she had only been to *parkrun* before as a spectator. In the past, she had watched with her grandmother as her parents took part, but on this occasion – and like so many youngsters in her shoes – she wanted to join in.

'Are you having fun?' I asked.

'We both are.' The girl's grandmother was wearing a pair of trainers that looked like they'd been borrowed for the morning, but I didn't want to ask. 'It's an adventure.'

We took the best part of an hour to reach the finish line. In that time, as the girl went on a mission to count the clouds in the sky, her grandmother told me that for various reasons life had not been easy for the family. She didn't need to go into detail, but I sensed that just talking with someone who had the time to listen was enough. As we approached course signage at various turns, I pretended that I didn't know the way to much laughter from the little girl. Under her direction and endless chatter, we all had a great time. Wearing her orange bib, even the tail-walker joined us on the final stretch, which signalled to the timekeepers as we came within sight of the finishing funnel that nobody else was behind her.

Catching sight of her parents among the throng of finishers, the little girl scampered the last few metres, but not so fast as to miss out on a high-five from each timekeeper. It was a lovely moment and one of countless others in a worldwide community that had grown beyond anything I could have imagined when I started something just to make a few friends. In October 2024, *parkrun* celebrated its twentieth anniversary. Even with an incredible 10 million registered participants, and a weekly average of 300,000 taking part in over 2,000 events across 23 countries, I still can't help feeling like it's a milestone on a greater journey. There are more than 8 billion people on earth, after all. Sometimes I wonder how life would be if every human being had access to a *parkrun* in their community. It might seem out of reach, but then look how far we've come.

'I can't believe we've done it,' said my walking companion, who had expressed some doubt that she and her granddaughter would be capable of completing the course. There was no obligation on anyone to go all the way. If it proved too much they could always come back and try again. All the same, I just encouraged her to just take it at her own pace. Now we had arrived at the end, and she could not have been more surprised at what she'd achieved.

'Your first *parkrun*,' I said, smiling at both timekeepers. 'Hopefully the first of many.'

On the other side of the funnel, having collected her finish token, the little girl had joined her mum and dad. In her father's arms, she was no doubt recounting every last conversation we'd just shared. Having clearly enjoyed a little break from their relentless offspring, and even some time together, both parents looked recharged and ready for the day.

'Thank you,' said the girl's grandmother. 'From us all.'

'It's been my pleasure,' I said, as we finished along with the tail-walker to bring everyone safely home. 'I enjoyed every step of the way.'

THE END

Acknowledgements

There are too many people to name who have touched my life during the making of *parkrun*. You know who you are. Thank you for taking the time to share your story with me, to influence the direction of my day and for putting a smile on my face.

To my wife, Joanne, thank you. She was there at the start and will be at the finish too. Constant throughout. Bringing sanity to my day. Joanne has helped correct the most obvious mistakes I have made in this book. Some may remain.

Surprisingly, but with full acceptance, our children haven't made *parkrun* their home yet but have been along for the ride. It's been a pleasure sharing the journey with you Morgan, Matthew, Jo, Ruby and Dylan.

Our grandsons, Solly and Caleb are toying with the idea of becoming parkrunners and we are watching very carefully.

Duncan Gaskell and Jim Desmond: Supporters, encouragers and friends. They challenged me when it was needed.

Ray and Ann Coward: The first Event Directors. Friends and *parkrun* champions. The T-shirt pixies. If you know then you know.

Chris Wright: He made a significant contribution to steering the ship in the early days and *parkrun* wouldn't be what it is without him.

Anita Pellew: Our second employee and the founder of *parkrun* France. A force for good, with incredible dedication and courage in the early years and remains a supporter. We were always loved and supported by Alex, Sofia and Eva too.

Richard Leyton, Alan Dempster and Jane Niven: IT wizards that turned a hobby IT system into a professional system. Also Orlando Pelicano & Steve McClune helped process the results and offered many good ideas for improvement.

Stuart Lodge: Always a supporter and often a mentor, created the clever linking capability in our results system and the inspiration for the name '*parkrun*'.

The *parkrun* pioneers: Those folks who came to the first event to run and volunteer when nobody knew what it would become, all of whom have gone onto great heights in their running careers. Chris, Matthew, John, Andrew, Steve, Peter, Rachel, James, Rachel, Karen, Julie, Tanya and Simon and volunteers Robin, Duncan, Joanne and Simon. Other pioneers followed with the internationalization of *parkrun*: Jonathan Sydenham, Tim Oberg, Rick Brauer, Matt & Ruth Shields, Bruce & Gill Fordyce, Noel & Lian DeCharmoy, Richard McChesney and Anita Pellew.

Nick Read: A believer on a similar journey. He has supported *parkrun* through thick and thin and remains a pillar for *parkrun*.

Hugh Brasher: Supported *parkrun* and me from the outset. Always challenged me.

London Marathon Foundation, Nick Bitel and David Bedford: Without their support, we might not have made it.

Nick Pearson: He stepped in to do a job I was no longer able to do.

Tom Williams: Nearly killed me but in the process drove professional standards in operations to maturity.

Russ Jefferys: Our current CEO, steadied the ship while driving the charity mission and purpose with pride and humility.

Our Trustee Board: Past and present. Always there, never acknowledged, driving standards throughout. Loyal supporters and champions of *parkrun*. Special mention to Christine Gibbons and Jeremy Townsend who have consistently contributed throughout. I'd also like to mention Andrew Lane who supported me from day one, encouraged The Stragglers Running Club to embrace *parkrun* and served as a trustee before accepting a role as an ambassador.

Thank you to our staff, past and present, across the world whose job it is to bring the movement to those who most need it. Unsung heroes and for the most part hidden. Your work is vital.

Every person who ever volunteered and those who are yet to discover the joy of volunteering. A special thanks to the event teams and ambassadors who trod a similar path to that which I walked. You are all game changers in your communities. You uphold our mission.

There have been many thousands of individuals who offered their thoughts, ideas and suggestions over the years, some of which found their way into the *parkrun* processes and procedures. Two examples of this are the Junior *parkrun* and the *parkrun* in the Custodial Estate programme. Paul Graham sought to introduce a *parkrun*, especially for juniors and Shane Spencer inspired the prison programme. Both initiatives have been enormously successful in delivering huge health benefits. Contributions have been made by many people over time for which I am eternally grateful.

While this book doesn't mention the many friends that I have met during my *parkrun* journey, I remain grateful for their love and support along the way. You contribute daily to my improved health and happiness.

And finally, I met Matt Whyman by pure chance. Having wrestled with the idea of writing a book for about ten years, Matt's wife, Emma, arrived in my life through the introduction of their dog Sprint. Sprint became a part of our extended family which led to meeting and getting to know the whole Whyman family. When you are unfamiliar with writing books, there are many pitfalls. Matt steered me through this process and also introduced me to my brilliant agent Ben Clark at The Soho Agency. My thanks to them all.

Pan Macmillan, managed by my editor Lydia Ramah, have been exceptional. Every interaction has been positive, encouraging, professional and focused. What's more, all the team have their own *parkrun* story to tell. Lucy Hale, Stuart Dwyer, Jo Mower, Mike Harpley, Jamie Forrest, Dylan van Dongen, Maddie Hanson, Rosie Shackles, Jenny Shone, Holly Sheldrake, Josie Turner, Katy Denny, Lucy Doncaster, Ross Jamieson, Sam Burt, Andy Joannou, Josie Turner.

I have so much to be thankful for.